Prevention
of Intimate Partner Violence

Prevention of Intimate Partner Violence has been co-published simultaneously as *Journal of Aggression, Maltreatment & Trauma*, Volume 13, Numbers 3/4, 2006.

Monographic Separates from the *Journal of Aggression, Maltreatment & Trauma*™

For additional information on these and other Haworth Press titles, including descriptions, tables of contents, reviews, and prices, use the QuickSearch

Prevention of Intimate Partner Violence, edited by Sandra M. Stith, PhD (Vol. 13, No. 3/4, 2006). *A comprehensive overview of effective approaches in working to prevent intimate partner violence.*

Ending Child Abuse: New Efforts in Prevention, Investigation, and Training, edited by Victor I. Vieth, JD, BS, Bette L. Bottoms, PhD, Alison R. Perona, JD, MA, BS (Vol. 12, No. 3/4, 2006).*A collection of innovative approaches and aggressive strategies to end or significantly reduce child abuse in every community.*

Trauma Treatment Techniques: Innovative Trends, edited by Jacueline Garrick, CSW, ACSW, BCETS, and Mary Beth Williams, PhD, LSW, CTS (Vol. 12, No. 1/2, 2006). *"This collection SIGNIFICANTLY BROADENS THE UNDERSTANDING OF INNOVATIVE TECHNIQUES for the treatment of PTSD and associated conditions." (John P. Wilson, Co-founder and Past President, International Society for Traumatic Stress Studies, Co-director, International Institute on Psychotraumatology)*

Ethical and Legal Issues for Mental Health Professionals: A Comprehensive Handbook of Principles and Standards, edited by Steven F. Bucky, Joanne E. Callan, and George Stricker (Vol. 11, No. 1/2 and 3, 2005). *"It is safe to say that every psychotherapist will be confronted with ethical and legal problems in the course of his or her career. THIS BOOK SHOULD BE RETAINED ON THE SHELF OF EVERY MENTAL HEALTH PRACTITIONER. This is an exhaustive compendium written by a distinguished battery of attorneys and psychotherapists, each of whom is an expert in his or her field . . . . It should be used as a resource guide when problems arise in the course of one's practice." (Martin Fleishman, MD, PhD, Active Staff, St. Francis Memorial Hospital, San Francisco; Author of "The Casebook of Residential Care Psychiatrist")*

The Trauma of Terrorism: Sharing Knowledge and Shared Care, An International Hanbook, edited by Yael Danieli, PhD, Danny Brom, PhD, and Joe Sills, MA (Vol. 9, No. 1/2 and 3/4, 2004 and Vol. 10, No. 1/2 and 3/4, 2005. *"This book pulls together key programs that enable society to cope with ongoing terrorism, and its thus a rich resource for both policymakers and those who aid terrorism's victims directly. It demonstrates the invaluable collaboration between government and private initiative in the development of a resilient society." (Danny Naveh, Minister of Health, Government of Israel)*

The Victimization of Children: Emerging Issues, edited by Janet L. Mullings, PhD, James W. Marquart, PhD, and Deborah J. Hartley, MS (Vol. 8, No. 1/2 [#15/16] and 3 [#17], 2003). *"A fascinating, illuminating, and often troubling collection of research on child victimization, abuse, and neglect. This book . . . is timely, thought-provoking, and an important contribution to the literature. No other book on the market today provides such an authoritative overview of the complex issues involved in child victimization." (Craig Hemmens, JD, PhD, Chair and Associate Professor, Department of Criminal Justice Administration, Boise State University)*

Intimate Violence: Contemporary Treatment Innovations, edited by Donald Dutton, PhD, and Daniel J. Sonkin, PhD (Vol. 7, No. 1/2 [#13/14], 2003). *"Excellent. . . . Represents 'outside the box' thinking. I highly recommend this book for everyone working in the field of domestic violence who wants to stay fresh. Readers will be stimulated and in most cases very valuably informed." (David B. Wexler, PhD, Executive Director, Relationship Training Institute, San Diego, CA)*

Trauma and Juvenile Delinquency: Theory, Research, and Interventions, edited by Ricky Greenwald, PsyD (Vol. 6, No. 1 [#11], 2002). *"Timely, concise, compassionate, and stimulating. . . . An impressive array of authors deals with various aspects of the problem in depth. This book will be of considerable interest to clinicians, teachers, and researchers in the mental health field, as well as administrators and juvenile justice personnel handling juvenile delinquents. I highly commend Dr. Greenwald on a job well done." (Hans Steiner, MD, Professor of Psychiatry and Behavioral Sciences, Stanford University School of Medicine)*

Domestic Violence Offenders: Current Interventions, Research, and Implications for Policies and Standards, edited by Robert Geffner, PhD, and Alan Rosenbaum, PhD (Vol. 5, No. 2 [#10], 2001).

The Shaken Baby Syndrome: A Multidisciplinary Approach, edited by Stephen Lazoritz, MD, and Vincent J. Palusci, MD (Vol. 5, No. 1 [#9], 2001). *The first book to cover the full spectrum of Shaken Baby Syndrome (SBS). Offers expert information and advice on every aspect of prevention, diagnosis, treatment, and follow-up.*

Trauma and Cognitive Science: A Meeting of Minds, Science, and Human Experience, edited by Jennifer J. Freyd, PhD, and Anne P. DePrince, MS (Vol. 4, No. 2 [#8] 2001). *"A fine collection of scholarly works that address key questions about memory for childhood and adult traumas from a variety of disciplines and empirical approaches. A must-read volume for anyone wishing to understand traumatic memory." (Kathryn Quina, PhD, Professor of Psychology & Women's Studies, University of Rhode Island)*

Program Evaluation and Family Violence Research, edited by Sally K. Ward, PhD, and David Finkelhor, PhD (Vol. 4, No. 1 [#7], 2000). *"Offers wise advice to evaluators and others interested in understanding the impact of their work. I learned a lot from reading this book." (Jeffrey L. Edleson, PhD, Professor, University of Minnesota, St. Paul)*

Sexual Abuse Litigation: A Practical Resource for Attorneys, Clinicians, and Advocates, edited by Rebecca Rix, MALS (Vol. 3, No. 2 [#6], 2000). *"An interesting and well developed treatment of the complex subject of child sexual abuse trauma. The merger of the legal, psychological, scientific and historical expertise of the authors provides a unique, in-depth analysis of delayed discovery in CSA litigation. This book, including the extremely useful appendices, is a must for the attorney or expert witness who is involved in the representation of survivors of sexual abuse." (Leonard Karp, JD, and Cheryl L. Karp, PhD, co-authors, Domestic Torts: Family Violence, Conflict and Sexual Abuse)*

Prevention
of Intimate Partner Violence

Sandra M. Stith, PhD
Editor

Prevention of Intimate Partner Violence has been co-published simultaneously as *Journal of Aggression, Maltreatment & Trauma*, Volume 13, Numbers 3/4, 2006

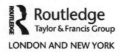

Routledge
Taylor & Francis Group

LONDON AND NEW YORK

Transferred to Digital Printing 2008 by Routledge 2008
2 Park Square, Milton Park, Abingdon, Oxon, OX14 4RN
270 Madison Ave, New York NY 10016

Published by

The Haworth Maltreatment & Trauma Press, 10 Alice Street, Binghamton, NY 13904-1580 USA

The Haworth Maltreatment & Trauma Press is an imprint of The Haworth Press, Inc., 10 Alice Street, Binghamton, NY 13904-1580 USA.

Prevention of Intimate Partner Violence has been co-published simultaneously as *Journal of Aggression, Maltreatment & Trauma*, Volume 13, Numbers 3/4 2006.

The development, preparation, and publication of this work has been undertaken with great care. However, the publisher, employees, editors, and agents of The Haworth Press and all imprints of The Haworth Press, Inc., including The Haworth Medical Press® and The Pharmaceutical Products Press®, are not responsible for any errors contained herein or for consequences that may ensue from use of materials or information contained in this work. The Haworth Press is committed to the dissemination of ideas and information according to the highest standards of intellectual freedom and the free exchange of ideas. Statements made and opinions expressed in this publication do not necessarily reflect the views of the Publisher, Directors, management, or staff of The Haworth Press, Inc., or an endorsement by them.

Cover design by Kerry E. Mack

Library of Congress Cataloging-in-Publication Data

Prevention of intimate partner violence / Sandra M. Stith, editor.
     p. cm.– (Journal of aggression, maltreatment & trauma monographic "separates")
     "Prevention of intimate partner violence has been co-published simultaneously as Journal of aggression, maltreatment & trauma, Volume 13, numbers 3/4 2006."
     Includes bibliographical references and index.
     ISBN 10: 0-7890-3032-2 (hard cover: alk. paper)
     ISBN 13: 978-0-7890-3032-0 (hard cover: alk. paper)
     ISBN 10: 0-7890-3033-0 (soft cover: alk. paper)
     ISBN 13: 978-0-7890-3033-7 (hard cover: alk. paper)
     1. Marital violence–United States. 2. Marital violence–United States–Prevention. I. Stith, Sandra M. II. Series: Journal of aggression, maltreatment & trauma.
HV6626.2.P74 2006
362.82'927–dc22
                                                  2005014036

Indexing, Abstracting & Website/Internet Coverage

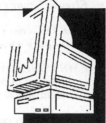

Journal of Aggression, Maltreatment & Trauma

This section provides you with a list of major indexing & abstracting services and other tools for bibliographic access. That is to say, each service began covering this periodical during the year noted in the right column. Most Websites which are listed below have indicated that they will either post, disseminate, compile, archive, cite or alert their own Website users with research-based content from this work. (This list is as current as the copyright date of this publication.)

Abstracting, Website/Indexing Coverage . . . . Year When Coverage Began

- *Cambridge Scientific Abstracts (A leading publisher of scientific information in print journals, online databases, CD-ROM and via the Internet) <http://www.csa.com>* 1997

- *Child Welfare Information Gateway (formerly National Adoption Information Clearinghouse Documents Database, and formerly National Adoption Information Clearinghouse on Child Abuse & Neglect Information Documents Database) <http://www.childwelfare.gov>* 2006

- *CINAHL (Cumulative Index to Nursing & Allied Health Literature), (EBSCO) <http://www.cinahl.com>* 2000

- *Criminal Justice Abstracts* 1997

- *EBSCOhost Electronic Journals Service (EJS) <http://ejournals.ebsco.com>* 2001

- *Educational Administration Abstracts (Sage)* 2001

- *Elsevier Eflow-I* 2006

(continued)

(continued)

(continued)

*Special Bibliographic Notes related to special journal issues
(separates) and indexing/abstracting:*

- indexing/abstracting services in this list will also cover material in any "separate" that is co-published simultaneously with Haworth's special thematic journal issue or DocuSerial. Indexing/abstracting usually covers material at the article/chapter level.
- monographic co-editions are intended for either non-subscribers or libraries which intend to purchase a second copy for their circulating collections.
- monographic co-editions are reported to all jobbers/wholesalers/approval plans. The source journal is listed as the "series" to assist the prevention of duplicate purchasing in the same manner utilized for books-in-series.
- to facilitate user/access services all indexing/abstracting services are encouraged to utilize the co-indexing entry note indicated at the bottom of the first page of each article/chapter/contribution.
- this is intended to assist a library user of any reference tool (whether print, electronic, online, or CD-ROM) to locate the monographic version if the library has purchased this version but not a subscription to the source journal.
- individual articles/chapters in any Haworth publication are also available through the Haworth Document Delivery Service (HDDS).

ABOUT THE EDITOR

Sandra M. Stith, PhD, is Professor and Director of the Marriage and Family Therapy program at Virginia Tech's Northern Virginia Campus in Falls Church, VA. Dr. Stith is a licensed Marriage and Family Therapist. She facilitated a support group at a shelter for battered women for several years and has provided treatment to victims, offenders, and couples wanting to end intimate partner violence. Dr. Stith's primary research interest is in the area of partner violence. Dr. Stith is a co-editor of two books on domestic violence: *Understanding Partner Violence: Prevalence, Causes, Consequences and Solutions* (1995), co-edited with Dr. Murray Straus and *Violence Hits Home: Comprehensive Treatment Approaches to Domestic Violence* (1990), co-edited with Drs. Mary Beth Williams and Karen Rosen. She is author of over 50 articles and book chapters published in a variety of journals including: *Journal of Marital and Family Therapy, Journal of Social and Personal Relationships, Family Relations, Journal of Family Violence, Violence and Victims, Aggression and Violent Behavior, Journal of Interpersonal Violence,* and *Journal of Marriage and the Family.* She received funding for her work developing a couples' treatment program for intimate partner violence from the National Institute of Mental Health. Dr. Stith has also received funding from the Family Advocacy Programs of each U.S. military branch to develop and pilot test risk assessment tools for intimate partner violence and child maltreatment. She has presented widely both nationally and internationally in the area of intimate partner violence. Dr. Stith is an active member of the National Council on Family Relations, the American Family Therapy Association, and the American Association for Marriage and Family Therapy and served on its Commission on Accreditation for Family Therapy Education for six years. She is the recipient of the 2004 American Association for Marriage and Family Therapy Outstanding Contribution to Marriage and Family Therapy Award.

Prevention
of Intimate Partner Violence

CONTENTS

About the Contributors

Gary L. Bowen, PhD, is Kenan Distinguished Professor in the School of Social Work at the University of North Carolina at Chapel Hill. He also holds a joint appointment in the Department of Communication Studies at the University of North Carolina at Chapel Hill, and is a Spencer Program Faculty Member, Spencer Foundation Education Policy Research Training Program, at Duke University. He is a Fellow of the National Council on Family Relations. Dr. Boen received the "Most Innovative Professor Award" in 2002 from the Social Work Student Organization at the University of North Carolina at Chapel Hill.

Jacquelyn Campbell, PhD, RN, is the Anna D. Wolf Chair and Associate Dean for Faculty Affairs in the Johns Hopkins University School of Nursing with a joint appointment in the Bloomberg School of Public Health. Her BSN, MSN, and PhD are from Duke University, Wright State University, and the University of Rochester. She has been conducting advocacy policy work and research in the area of domestic violence since 1980. Dr. Campbell has been the PI of 9 major NIH, NIJ, or CDC research grants, and has published more than 125 articles and 6 books on this subject. She is an elected member of the Institute of Medicine and the American Academy of Nursing and on the Boards of Directors of the Family Violence Prevention Fund and the House of Ruth Battered Women's Shelter, and was a member of the congressionally appointed US Department of Defense Task Force on Domestic Violence.

Patti A. T. Fritz, MA, is a doctoral candidate in clinical psychology at Stony Brook University. Her research interests include the etiology, prevention, and treatment of interpersonal aggression with specific emphases on individuals' attributions about their use of partner aggression, contextual factors surrounding partner aggression, and the stability of partner aggression across time and generations. She has collaborated on a number of projects exploring the longitudinal course of interpersonal aggression and has assisted in the evaluation of aggression prevention and intervention programs for youth. She has published in *Violence and Victims*, and has presented her findings at such conferences as the Society for Research in Child Development, the Association for the Advancement of Behavior Therapy, and the International Family Research Violence Conference.

L. Kevin Hamberger, PhD, is Professor of Family and Community Medicine in the Department of Family and Community Medicine, Medical College of Wisconsin. Since 1982, he has conducted treatment and research programs with domestically violent men and women, and developed and evaluated health care provider training programs to deliver violence prevention services to patients. Dr. Hamberger is Co-Chair of the Wisconsin Governor's Council for Domestic Abuse and founding member and past Chair of the Wisconsin Batterer Treatment Provider Association. He has served as a consultant to the National Institutes of Health, National Institute of Mental Health, the National Institute of Justice, the Department of Defense, and the Family Violence Prevention Fund. He is on the editorial boards of 4 scholarly journals. Dr. Hamberger has published approximately 80 articles, chapters and 5 books, including *Treating Men Who Batter: Theories, Programs, and Practice* (Springer), *Domestic Partner Abuse* (Springer), and *Violence Issues for Health Care Educators and Providers* (The Haworth Press, Inc.)

Sherry L. Hamby, PhD, is Research Associate Professor at the University of North Carolina at Chapel Hill. She is co-author of *The Conflict Tactics Scales* handbook, and author or co-author of more than 30 other publications on family violence and assessment. She has received the Wellner Memorial Award from the National Register for Health Service Providers in Psychology. She is currently vice president of the board of her local domestic violence shelter. Recently, she helped adapt a partner violence prevention program for French-speaking Switzerland. Other interests include the measurement of violence, American Indian communities, and the use of qualitative techniques to address persistent controversies in partner violence research.

David W. Lloyd, JD, is Director of the Family Advocacy Program in the Office of the Secretary of Defense, responsible for policy development and budget support of the social services programs in the Military Departments that address the prevention, intervention, and treatment of child abuse and domestic violence at military installations worldwide.

He was previously the Director of the National Center on Child Abuse and Neglect, in the U.S. Department of Health and Human Services. He has conducted training at numerous national conferences on family violence and has also written extensively on child maltreatment in professional books and journals.

Jay A. Mancini, PhD, is Professor of Human Development at Virginia Polytechnic Institute and State University, Blacksburg, VA. He received his doctoral degree in family studies from the University of North Carolina at Greensboro, and received UNC-G's 2002 Human Environmental Science Distinguished Alumnus Award. His research focuses on lifespan human development, the sustainability of community-based programs, building community capacity, and on military families. Dr. Mancini is a Fellow of the National Council on Family Relations.

Jennifer Manganello, PhD, MPH, has been a Post-Doctoral Research Fellow at the Annenberg Public Policy Center, University of Pennsylvania, since July of 2003. Before coming to Annenberg, Dr. Manganello earned her PhD from the Department of Health Policy and Management at the Johns Hopkins Bloomberg School of Public Health. While at Johns Hopkins, Dr. Manganello was a Pre-Doctoral Fellow with the Interdisciplinary Research Training on Violence grant awarded by the National Institute of Mental Health. Her dissertation research examined violence against women and health care policy issues in the news. Dr. Manganello has participated in research studies related to the prevention of violence against women and the improvement of health outcomes for children. Prior to attending Johns Hopkins, Dr. Manganello worked at the Institute for Health Policy Research at Massachusetts General Hospital in Boston for three years. She earned a BA from Pomona College and an MPH from Boston University.

James A. Martin, PhD, BCD, Colonel, U.S. Army (Retired) is a faculty member in the Graduate School of Social Work and Social Research at Bryn Mawr College. A Licensed Independent Clinical Social Worker and a Board Certified Diplomate in Clinical Social Work, he regularly teaches courses in clinical social work practice and human services program management and evaluation. Dr. Martin's practice and scholarship focuses on issues related to human services, military family issues, and the development of 21st century military communities.

John P. Nelson, PhD, Colonel, USAF (Retired) is a consultant with particular interests in areas of community enhancement, military family issues and youth development. Dr. Nelson's current work is focused on community building initiatives and collaboration across human-service agencies. He holds a PhD in Social Work from the University of Minnesota, and was the recipient of the 2001-2002 National Partner-in-4H Award, the highest public award conferred by the 4-H program.

K. Daniel O'Leary, PhD, is Distinguished Professor of Psychology and past Chairman of the Psychology Department at Stony Brook University. O'Leary was among the top 100 cited psychologists in the English-speaking world (*American Psychologist*, December, 1978). He received the Distinguished Scientist Award from the clinical division of the American Psychological Association in 1985, and he was installed to the National Academies of Practice in Psychology in 1986. He is the author or co-author of ten books. The most recent include: *The Couples Psychotherapy Treatment Planner* with R. E. Heyman and A. E. Jongsma (1998), and *Psychological Abuse in Violent Domestic Relations* (with R.D. Maiuro, 2001). His research focuses on the etiology and treatment of partner aggression, and the marital discord/depression link.

Mary Beth Phelan, MD, is a board-certified Associate Professor of Emergency Medicine in the Department of Emergency Medicine, Medical College of Wisconsin. Her major areas of interest are domestic violence and ultrasonography. Dr. Phelan completed an Emergency Ultrasound fellowship in 1994, and has contributed extensively to the advancement of emergency ultrasound through workshops and peer reviewed journal publications. Dr. Phelan also has worked in the area of intimate partner violence through development of emergency medicine training curricula, curricula evaluation, and research on male and female victims of intimate partner violence who seek emergency medical services. Additionally, she has contributed to development of domestic violence guidelines that were accepted by the Agency for Health Care Policy and Research's National Guideline Clearing House for Website publication.

Nancy Sugg MD, MPH, is Associate Professor of Medicine at the University of Washington and the Medical Director of the Pioneer Square Clinic in Seattle, Washington.

Erica M. Woodin, MA, is a doctoral candidate in clinical psychology at Stony Brook University, where she holds a Stony Brook Graduate Council Fellowship. Her research interests include the prevention and treatment of partner aggression and relationship distress, the prediction of relationship dissolution, and the examination of emotion and conflict in close relationships. She has collaborated on a number of projects exploring longitudinal trajectories and interventions for violent, distressed, and non-distressed couples, and is currently developing a brief motivational intervention for young adults experiencing low levels of physical aggression in their current dating relationships. She has published empirical articles in *Child Development, Journal of Family Communication,* and *Journal of Marital and Family Therapy*. She has also published a chapter documenting the need for integration of partner violence and child abuse prevention programs in an APA edited book, *Violence Prevention*.

Ricardo J. Wray, PhD, is Assistant Professor of Community Health at the Saint Louis University School of Public Health (SLU-SPH), where he teaches Communication. He is also a Principal Investigator at the Health Communication Research Laboratory at the SLU-SPH. As a doctoral student at the University of Pennsylvania, Dr. Wray took part in the development and evaluation of the Its Your Business project, a domestic violence prevention radio serial that sought to reach African Americans. His research elucidates the intersection of communication and public health, with an emphasis on public health theory and practice. In particular, his research seeks to understand: how communication efforts can overcome institutional, social and community level barriers to health care in the African American community; links between community-based health promotion and large-scale media efforts; and public health communication contributions to emergency response.

Foreword

The genesis for this volume is a 2002 Department of Defense (DoD) Symposium on Domestic Violence Prevention Research. Special thanks for this collection should therefore go to Sandra M. Stith, PhD, Program Director, Human Development Department, Virginia Polytechnic Institute and State University and to Lt. Col. Dari Tritt, USAF, BSC, both of whom took the major role in planning the 2002 Symposium. The 2002 Symposium brought together more than 40 domestic violence experts, researchers, and health care professionals from the Armed Forces, academia, and civilian governmental and nonprofit agencies to ascertain the empirical basis for policy and program development in the prevention of domestic violence, and to develop a research agenda for determining what will work in preventing domestic violence in the military community. Caliber Associates, Inc., of Fairfax, Virginia helped organize the Symposium and produced its final report.

The Symposium was part of a larger continuing DoD process to improve its response to domestic violence. In 1996 and 1997, the Deputy Assistant Secretary for Personnel Support, Families, and Education (now the Deputy Under Secretary of Defense for Military Community and Family Policy (DUSD[MC&FP]) sponsored a forum and a policy conference to assess intervention in domestic violence occurring in the military community and make recommendations for improving DoD's response. DoD has also benefited from the work of the Defense Task Force on Domestic Violence, which Congress authorized in 2000 and which concluded its work in 2003. Among the Task Force's recommendations to improve the DoD response to domestic violence were one that made an evaluation of prevention efforts a research priority and another that set forth a conceptual model for prevention approaches. The

[Haworth co-indexing entry note]: "Foreword." Lloyd, David W. Co-published simultaneously in *Journal of Aggression, Maltreatment & Trauma* (The Haworth Maltreatment & Trauma Press, an imprint of The Haworth Press, Inc.) Vol. 13, No. 3/4, 2006, pp. xxix-xxxi; and: *Prevention of Intimate Partner Violence* (ed: Sandra M. Stith) The Haworth Maltreatment & Trauma Press, an imprint of The Haworth Press, Inc., 2006, pp. xxi-xxiii. Single or multiple copies of this article are available for a fee from The Haworth Document Delivery Service [1-800-HAWORTH, 9:00 a.m. - 5:00 p.m. (EST). E-mail address: docdelivery@haworthpress.com].

DUSD (MC&FP) established an office that is implementing the Task Force's recommendations, and is already implementing both the number one research priority of the Symposium and a second research priority of the Task Force.

There are several reasons why DoD is particularly interested in preventing domestic violence. First, domestic violence is inconsistent with the core values of the military and it hurts morale. In addition, the active duty force is primarily composed of more than a million young adults, especially young adult males, which is demographically a high-risk group for a range of social problems, including interpersonal violence. About half of the active duty force is married, and DoD wants to have strong, violence-free marriages.

The second reason DoD is interested in preventing domestic violence is to reduce the costs that result from incidents of domestic violence. Domestic violence creates four cost areas to DoD: (a) the diminished military readiness of abusers; (b) the costs of law enforcement investigation, command personnel actions, legal proceedings under the Uniform Code of Military Justice, medical and supportive services to victims, and treatment services to abusers; (c) the cost of replacing those personnel separated from active duty due to domestic violence; and (d) transitional compensation, which is available to a family member who is the victim of child abuse or spouse abuse by a service member, when the service member is separated due to the abuse. The compensation is calculated based on the service member's pay and is for up to three years, depending on the amount of time remaining to the end of the service member's term. In addition, the victim is eligible for medical and dental benefits for a similar period of time. There are additional secondary cost areas to DoD, other governmental agencies, and the private sector that result from the costs of domestic violence: depression and related substance abuse, unemployment, and lost tax revenue from poor productivity.

The third reason DoD wants to prevent domestic violence is its generational impact. Experiencing abuse in childhood and witnessing violence in the family in childhood are risk factors for domestic violence in adulthood. In career active duty military families, there are more than 150,000 adolescents, and DoD wants to ensure that these teens have positive relationships in their families and dating relationships. Furthermore, DoD will draw nearly half its recruits from such young men and women who grew up in career active duty military families. In studies conducted for the Army and Navy, approximately a third of new recruits had experienced or witnessed family violence in childhood. If DoD can prevent violence in military families, a significant proportion of its next generation of recruits will be at lower risk for inflicting or experiencing domestic violence.

Although the Symposium was oriented to the military community, the Symposium planners and participants were always cognizant of the interest of the larger civilian community in domestic violence prevention research. This issue reflects the adaptation and expansion of the Symposium's papers and final report for the civilian context.

David W. Lloyd, JD
Director, Family Advocacy Program
Office of the Deputy Under Secretary of Defense
(Military Community & Family Policy)

Acknowledgments

This volume would not have been possible without the contribution of others. First, I want to acknowledge the contribution of Lieutenant Colonel Dari Tritt, USAF (ret), who contributed to every step of the project. She helped select the authors, coordinated the contributions, and helped with the first review of manuscripts. The collection would not have been possible without her contribution and the commitment and assistance to the project of the Air Force Family Advocacy Program and its former director, Colonel John Nelson, USAF (ret), BSC; and the Office of the Deputy Assistant Secretary of Defense for Military Community and Family Policy and, in particular, its Director of Family Advocacy Programs, Dr. David W. Lloyd. I also want to acknowledge the contributions of the authors of each manuscript and the attendees of the Department of Defense sponsored symposium on the Prevention of Intimate Partner Violence who contributed to developing the research suggestions presented in the final article in this publication. Finally, I want to thank Ms. Maggie Harris, who helped manage the process of editing the work and Jennifer Zellner and Bob Geffner for their guidance throughout the project.

Acknowledgements

Introduction

Sandra M. Stith, PhD

SUMMARY. This collection is an outgrowth of a symposium the Department of Defense held in May 2002 to develop a research agenda focusing on prevention of intimate partner violence. Subject area experts were asked to review the current literature on various aspects of intimate partner violence prevention in four primary areas, including what we know about: (a) changing the way people think about intimate partner violence; (b) changing the way the health care system responds to intimate partner violence; (c) changing the way young people handle anger and interact with their intimate partners; and (d) changing the ways communities support families to prevent intimate partner violence. In this volume, we compile the work of these scholars to further intervention and research efforts to prevent intimate partner violence. doi:10.1300/J146v13n03_01 *[Article copies available for a fee from The Haworth Document Delivery Service: 1-800-HAWORTH. E-mail address: <docdelivery@haworthpress.com> Website: <http://www.HaworthPress.com> © 2006 by The Haworth Press, Inc. All rights reserved.]*

KEYWORDS. Intimate partner violence, prevention, health care screening, media, community resilience

---

Address correspondence to Sandra M. Stith, PhD, 7054 Haycock Road, Falls Church, VA 22043 (E-mail: sstith@vt.edu).

[Haworth co-indexing entry note]: "Introduction." Stith, Sandra M. Co-published simultaneously in *Journal of Aggression, Maltreatment & Trauma* (The Haworth Maltreatment & Trauma Press, an imprint of The Haworth Press, Inc.) Vol. 13, No. 3/4, 2006, pp. 1-12; and: *Prevention of Intimate Partner Violence* (ed: Sandra M. Stith) The Haworth Maltreatment & Trauma Press, an imprint of The Haworth Press, Inc., 2006, pp. 1-12. Single or multiple copies of this article are available for a fee from The Haworth Document Delivery Service [1-800-HAWORTH, 9:00 a.m. - 5:00 p.m. (EST). E-mail address: docdelivery@haworthpress.com].

Available online at http://jamt.haworthpress.com
© 2006 by The Haworth Press, Inc. All rights reserved.
doi:10.1300/J146v13n03_01

INTRODUCTION

Intimate partner violence is a pervasive social problem that has devastating effects on all family members as well as on the larger community. Department of Justice Statistics indicate that the incidence of intimate partner violence is about 1 million cases per year for women and 150,000 cases per year for men (Rennison & Welchans, 2000). During the past 20 years, research on offenders and victims, risk factors for intimate partner violence, and on treatment of intimate partner violence has flourished. However, research on the prevention of intimate partner violence is still in its infancy.

While preventing interpersonal violence is the central goal of most intervention strategies, most programs and services are reactive by design. Some form of abuse must be substantiated or suspected before most services can be offered (Kurst-Swanger & Petcosky, 2003). In fact, Chalk and King (1998), in the National Research Council's publication, *Violence in Families: Assessing Prevention and Treatment Programs*, indicated that, "In all areas of family violence, after-the-fact services predominate over preventive interventions. . . . For domestic violence, interventions designed to treat victims and offenders and deter future incidents of violence are more common, but preventive services remain relatively underdeveloped" (p. 291). Even the field of health care still only designates 1% of health care spending to prevention efforts (Kurst-Swanger & Petcosky). Scarce resources, along with an ample number of identified abuse cases, lead decision makers to continue to fund programs dealing with the identified problems. Few resources are left to target a problem that may never come to be. While preventive services remain undeveloped, research on the effectiveness of these efforts is woefully lacking. The articles published in this volume review the published literature on prevention of intimate partner violence and suggest future directions for intervention and research in this area.

This collection is an outgrowth of a symposium the Department of Defense held in May 2002 to develop a research agenda focusing on prevention of intimate partner violence. Subject area experts were asked to review the current literature on various aspects of intimate partner violence prevention in four primary areas, including what we know about: (a) changing the way people think about intimate partner violence; (b) changing the way the health care system responds to intimate partner violence; (c) changing the way young people handle anger and interact with their intimate partners; and (d) changing the ways communities support families to prevent intimate partner violence. They were then asked to identify gaps in the research and cutting edge intervention and research issues. These authors and other researchers with recognized expertise in intimate partner violence, practitioners, and representatives from the Department of Defense and other federal agencies were asked to participate in working groups during the three-day symposium. Each working group developed a research plan to build on existing research and developed outlines of research projects that should be conducted to further the research in this area. This publication includes revised versions of each manuscript written for the symposium. The final article summarizes suggestions made by article authors and other participants in the symposium to guide future intimate partner violence prevention research efforts in each area.

This collection has several goals. First, we hope to inform prevention specialists about what is known about the effectiveness of various prevention interventions. By reviewing what is known about the effectiveness of current prevention programs, we hope that this volume will encourage prevention specialists to make use of evidence-based interventions in their own work. We also hope to encourage practitioners to become involved in evaluating the effectiveness of the work they are doing to prevent intimate partner violence. Finally, we also hope to foster more and better research into the prevention of intimate partner violence.

WHY FOCUS ON PREVENTION OF INTIMATE PARTNER VIOLENCE?

Most of the expanding body of intimate partner violence research has focused on clearly identifying the extent of the problem, defining the at-risk population or typologies within this population, and understanding the impact of the problem on its victims. Recent research has also focused on evaluating the effectiveness of various interventions, including criminal justice, legal, and therapeutic, in preventing the recurrence of the problem. However, a "growing frustration with the limitations of therapeutic interventions, and a clearer articulation of the costs that violence imposes on the wider society have all contributed to more robust prevention policies" (Daro, Edleson, & Pinderhughes, 2004, p. 289). Such policies offer a much-needed alternative to the treatment paradigms and the over emphasis on prosecution and punishment. However, the resources that have been made available for these prevention programs have often been used to support programs and services without adequate evidence of the effectiveness of the program or without adequate infrastructure to evaluate their effectiveness (Guterman, 2004). Practitioners often view intervention research as cumbersome and expensive given the immediate demands for services. On the other hand, from a research standpoint, questions are left about the value of carrying out expensive programming without any evidence that the programs are actually effective in preventing intimate partner violence. Guterman argues that the tension between needs of practitioners, researchers, and policy makers instills healthy pressures in all directions. "For researchers, such pressures mandate that research activities ultimately should be 'in the service of service' and that their findings should be expedited to practitioners and policy makers, accessible, useful, and flexible. For practitioners and policy makers, they mandate that their real world strategies are rigorously grounded, optimally evaluated in an objective fashion, providing greater accountability to the public and target recipients" (p. 311).

While programs designed to prevent intimate partner violence are expanding, research on their effectiveness is often lacking. Much has been written about the limitations and challenges of conducting treatment outcome research (e.g., Babcock & La Taillade, 2000; Edleson & Tolman, 1992); however, at least treatment outcome researchers can gauge interventions to treat violence after it occurs in a straightforward way by measuring reductions in violent behavior (Guterman, 2004). Prevention researchers are challenged to measure the effectiveness of their interventions by determining if they are able to avert behaviors (occurring at a relatively low base rate) that have not yet occurred and thus are less readily observable. While the field struggles with determining if the interventions that have been developed are effective in preventing violence, we also need to be increasing our efforts to understand the components and characteristics of interventions that are most effective in changing violence-related attitudes, beliefs, behavioral intentions, or skills (Schewe, 2002). Thus, this volume examines what is known about effective interpersonal violence prevention programs and offers suggestions for future research.

THEORETICAL FRAMEWORK

Theoretical perspectives on intimate partner violence have shifted from single factor to multi-factor frameworks. These multi-factor frameworks suggest that intimate partner violence is not simply caused by any one factor, such as an individual's psychological dysfunction, but rather results from the interaction between various characteristics of individuals and their environment. Clearly, interventions designed to prevent intimate partner violence must also address multiple factors.

Dutton's (1995) nested ecological theory on partner violence has guided our thinking about interventions to prevent intimate partner violence. This theory examines four levels of factors relating to individual offenders and their environment. The *macrosystem*, the broadest level, includes general cultural values and beliefs. The second paper in this volume, written by Campbell and Manganello, and the third paper by Wray address the use of media and public awareness campaigns to prevent intimate partner violence. These campaigns are frequently designed to address broad cultural values and beliefs (i.e., macrosystem factors).

The *exosystem* level includes the individual's formal and informal social structures such as their community, friendships, work place, and formal institutions such as the medical system, that connect the individual and their family to the larger culture. The fourth paper by Hamberger and Phelan and the fifth paper by Sugg in this volume address the medical system and the eighth paper in this volume by Mancini, Nelson, Bowen, and Martin addresses the community's potential to prevent intimate partner violence. Each of these papers target exosystemic factors.

The *microsystem* level includes characteristics of the immediate setting in which the abuse takes place. In other words, family units, the antecedents of abuse, consequences of abuse, and relationship dynamics are all included in the microsystem. Finally, the *ontogentic* level is specific to the abuser's developmental history or what the abuser brings to the current relationship from their past. Risk factors included in the ontogentic level include the offender's characteristics that influence their response to stressors occurring at the microsystem and exosystem levels, thus including risk factors relating to learned behaviors, cognitions, and emotional responses to stressors. The sixth paper by O'Leary, Woodin, and Fritz and the seventh paper by Hamby in this volume address prevention programs designed to prevent young people from engaging in intimate partner violence. These interventions address factors at both the microsystem and ontogentic levels. In addition, media and educational campaigns discussed in the second and third paper in this volume are also frequently designed to provide education to influence individuals' cognitions and behaviors (ontogentic factors). Thus, we have included articles on prevention of intimate partner violence at each level of the nested ecological theory.

RISK FACTORS FOR INTIMATE PARTNER VIOLENCE

A large body of research has focused on gaining a greater understanding of risk factors associated with physical abuse perpetration and victimization. Risk factors are characteristics associated with an increased likelihood that a problem behavior will occur. Although the presence of one or more risk markers does not necessarily indicate that a causal relationship is present, the odds of an associated event are greater when one or more risk markers are present. Numerous risk factors have been found to be associated with partner violence. O'Leary, Woodin, and Fitz (this volume) discuss some of these factors. However, findings across studies are often contradictory, making it difficult to condense the information into a general scope of knowledge on the topic. The development of intervention and prevention programs necessitates an understanding of these risk factors so that these programs are designed to target these factors.

We recently completed a meta-analytic review designed to summarize data on intimate partner violence risk factors between the years of 1980 and 2000 (Stith, Smith, Penn, Ward, & Tritt, 2004). Meta-analysis is a statistical method for reviewing multiple studies across the relevant research literature and provides a method for comparison of separate studies made possible through the use of effect sizes. The effect size is a statistical representation of the strength of the relationship between two variables. Evidence from 85 studies was examined to identify risk factors most strongly related to intimate partner physical abuse perpetration and victimization. The studies produced 308 distinct effect sizes. Dutton's (1995) nested ecological theory on partner violence, described above, was used to guide our selection of variables to be examined. We were unable to find at least four studies with appropriate data to calculate any composite effect sizes for factors at the macrosystem level or composite effect sizes for a number of other offender-related risk factors (e.g., violent toward non-family members, pet abuse, controlling behaviors, stalking, prior criminal history, marital separation, offender accountability, and empathy). However, we were able to calculate composite effect sizes for 16 risk factors for perpetrating intimate partner violence. In the following section, we review the results of this meta-analysis.

Exosystem Risk Factors

In general, it appears that factors at this level were least strongly related to intimate partner violence. None of the exosystem risk factors were computed to be strong risk factors for spouse maltreatment. Four of the exosystem variables–being unemployed, having a lower income, having a younger age, and having a lower education–were weak but significant predictors of intimate partner violence. Life stress had a moderate effect on intimate partner violence. While all of these factors, except level of stress, were weak predictors of intimate partner violence, there is evidence that targeting prevention programming to young, unemployed, lower income individuals with a lower level of education and a higher level of stress might be most cost-effective. O'Leary, Woodin, and Fritz (this volume) discuss advantages of targeting prevention programs to at-risk groups versus providing universal prevention programming.

Microsystem Risk Factors

Risk factors at the microsystem level (i.e., those factors associated with direct interactions or contexts in which abuse occurs) are some of the most important risk markers for intimate physical abuse of a partner. In fact, the effect size for emotionally abusing a partner and for forcing a partner to have sex resulted in the two strongest effect sizes for current physical abuse of a partner. Having a past history of being physically abusive is a moderate correlate of current physical abuse. Low marital satisfaction is also a strong microsystem risk factor for men using physical violence and a moderate risk factor for women using physical violence against their partners. Excessive jealousy is a moderate predictor of men using physical violence against their partners. Risk factors at the microsystem level are most relevant for developing programs that target individuals who are in troubled relationships or where violence is already occurring (tertiary or indicated prevention). Couples counseling or premarital interventions can target individuals in conflictual relationships before violence has occurred.

Ontogentic Risk Factors

The effect sizes for ontogentic risk factors ranged from small to strong. Illicit drug use and having attitudes condoning violence are strong correlates of being physically abusive. Traditional sex-role ideology, high levels of anger/hostility, alcohol abuse, and depression are moderate risk factors for men using physical violence against their partners. Interventions designed to change public attitudes and individual behavior can be used to address these risk factors.

ARTICLES IN THIS VOLUME

As indicated, the articles in this volume address the issue of preventing intimate partner violence. We are interested in averting violent events before they occur. Guterman (2004) uses the public health terminology of *primary*, *secondary*, and *tertiary* prevention interventions, and the more recently proposed terms of *universal*, *selected*, and *indicated* prevention, to organize preventive principles and strategies under study. Primary prevention is proactive, in that it seeks to build strengths in normal populations to ward off maladaptive problems. Primary prevention programs, or universal prevention programs, refer to educational or media programs that target an entire community or social group. Public service announcements and dating violence prevention programs included in the curriculum for the entire school are examples of primary prevention programs. Secondary, or selected, prevention targets those identified as at-risk for developing certain kinds of problems (Low, Monarch, Hartman, & Markman, 2002). Secondary prevention involves identifying a high-risk sample of the population and providing interventions for this group. For example, since low marital satisfaction has been identified as a risk factor for intimate partner violence, programs that target couples in conflictual relationships would be considered secondary prevention efforts. Finally, tertiary, or indicated, prevention targets individuals who have already been violent and tries to stop future occurrences or relapses. Treatment for batterers is an example of tertiary prevention programs. Hamby (1998) suggests that the lines between these three kinds of prevention are often not razor sharp. For example, hospital intimate partner violence screening procedures may have the dual effect of reducing society's tolerance for partner violence (primary prevention) and providing resources to assist victims escape from violent relationships (tertiary prevention). Guterman argues, as do we, for the importance of distinguishing between prevention of violence before it occurs (largely, primary and secondary or universal and selected prevention), which is the focus of this volume, from 'after-the-fact treatment' (a.k.a., tertiary/indicated prevention), which falls outside the purview of this volume.

The articles in this volume describe state-of-the-art prevention programs for intimate partner violence. They address challenges of conducting and evaluating such programs, gaps in programming and research, and future trends in prevention programming and research. The areas selected for inclusion in this volume represented a multi-focal approach to intimate partner violence prevention. The book is divided into five sections. The first section addresses changing the ways individuals think about and respond to intimate partner violence. The second section focuses on changing the ways the health care system responds to intimate partner violence. The third section addresses changing the ways young people deal with anger and intimate partner relationships, and the fourth section addresses changing the ways society and especially the community supports families to reduce the occurrence of intimate partner violence. The final section of this volume summarizes recommendations for future research.

We first looked at media and public education campaigns as ways to influence individuals, institutions, and societal norms and expectations. Public education campaigns to prevent intimate partner violence have been used in several ways. First, these campaigns have been used to educate abused women about community resources, such as shelters, and about other strategies for getting help. They have also been used in an effort to encourage witnesses of intimate partner violence to get involved and provide support to victims or report abuse to criminal justice authorities. Finally, they have been used in an effort to change public attitudes and norms about intimate partner violence. The second article in this volume, by Campbell and Mangangello, reviews published research on public awareness campaigns regarding intimate partner violence and child abuse and discusses lessons learned from other health education campaigns, including anti-smoking campaigns, substance abuse campaigns, and HIV/AIDS campaigns. The authors discuss the potential for success and the limitations of this type of intervention and offer suggestions for developing more effective campaigns.

In the third article in this volume, Ricardo Wray expands on Campbell and Mangangello's paper from a communication theory perspective and focuses on the importance of theory in guiding media campaigns to prevent interpersonal violence. Dr. Wray argues that while theory and evidence are considered essential underpinnings for intervention design and assessment in research and practice in the broader context of health communication, campaigns that promote intimate partner violence prevention often make very little explicit or formal use of theory. He makes a strong case for the idea that without a clear theory about what causes interpersonal violence, it is unlikely we can be successful in developing interventions to prevent interpersonal violence. He offers concrete guidance on how to apply various theories in developing more effective media campaigns to prevent intimate partner violence.

The next area reviewed in this volume involves changing the way the health care system responds to intimate partner violence. In recent years, the prevention of intimate partner violence has become a national and international public health priority. Organizations such as the Centers for Disease Control and Prevention, the World Health Organization, the American Medical Association, and the American College of Emergency Physicians have issued strong policy statements regarding the priority of this issue. However, the authors of the fourth and fifth articles of this volume explain why health care settings have been slow to change the way they respond to intimate partner violence and offer suggestions for overcoming the barriers to change. First, in the fourth paper in this volume, Hamberger and Phelan argue that the patient-physician encounter has the potential to play a critical role in preventing future intimate partner violence; however, barriers exist to providing care to patients experiencing intimate partner violence. The authors review current research that evaluates physician, patient, and systems barriers to providing this care and offer suggestions for how these barriers might be overcome. Dr. Sugg, in the next article in this volume, clearly articulates what she believes is necessary for medical providers to accept intimate partner violence as a part of their professional purview and to be successful in intervening. She highlights the importance of presenting convincing data to medical personal as to the prevalence of intimate partner violence among their patients and the reasons that intimate partner violence should be conceptualized as a medical problem. She clearly articulates the need for a short, reliable assessment instrument and protocols that can be used by medical personnel to assess and intervene in intimate partner violence in a variety of medical settings. She addresses the question of the best way to educate medical personnel and to acquire institutional, professional association, and research support to galvanize the medical profession in its response to intimate partner violence.

The third section in this volume addresses how to change the ways young people deal with anger and intimate partner relationships. In their paper, O'Leary, Woodin, and Fritz provide an extensive review of intimate partner prevention programs targeting young adults. Because they found relatively few published prevention programs in this area, they also reviewed programs designed to reduce sexual aggression, substance abuse, and acting-out behavior in young adults–antisocial behaviors that often co-occur with partner aggression. Finally, they draw from all of this literature to present a tiered approach to the prevention of intimate partner violence. This model draws from primary, secondary, and tertiary prevention efforts to intervene with all individuals, moderate aggressors, and severe aggressors.

The second article addressing how to change the way young people deal with anger and intimate partner relationships was written by Hamby. She expands upon the previous article, which reviews the published research and suggests a tiered approach to prevention. Hamby articulates issues relevant for a coherent program of partner violence prevention research. These issues include the appropriate scope, format, audience, setting, and mechanics of partner violence prevention.

In the eighth article in this volume, Mancini and colleagues explore the importance of community-level interventions for preventing intimate partner violence. They argue for active, network-oriented prevention efforts. They present implications for program development that include community as a place for prevention, a target for prevention, and as a force for prevention. Implications for research include examining multiple community layers, the nexus of informal and formal social care systems, and contrasting extreme groups on pivotal social organization processes.

Together these papers point to an emerging research as well as practice and policy agenda to prevent intimate partner violence using a multi-factorial approach. The issues associated with intimate partner violence are far too complicated to be eliminated by any one specific prevention or intervention program, or even one type of program. A much broader range of prevention efforts is required. The articles in this volume advocate for collaborative, coordinated, multidisciplinary approaches to intimate partner violence prevention.

REFERENCES

Babcock, J. C., & La Taillade, J. J. (2000). Evaluating interventions for men who batter. In J. P. Vincent & E. N. Jouriles (Eds.), *Domestic violence: Guidelines for research-informed practice* (pp. 37-77). London: Jessica Kingsley.

Chalk, R., & King, P. (Eds.) (1998). *Violence in families: Assessing prevention and treatment programs.* Washington, DC: National Academy Press.

Daro, D., Edleson, J. L., & Pinderhughes, H. (2004). Finding common ground in the study of child maltreatment, youth violence, and adult domestic violence. *Journal of Interpersonal Violence, 19,* 282-298.

Dutton, D.G. (1995). The domestic assault of women: Psychological and criminal justice perspectives. Vancouver, British Columbia: UBC Press.

Edleson, J. L., & Tolman, R. M. (1992). *Intervention for men who batter: An ecological approach.* Thousand Oaks, CA: Sage.

Guterman, N. B. (2004). Advancing prevention research on child abuse, youth violence, and domestic violence: Emerging strategies and issues. *Journal of Interpersonal Violence, 19,* 299-321.

Hamby, S. L. (1998). Partner violence: Prevention and intervention. In J. L. Jasinski & L. M. Williams (Eds.), Partner *violence: A comprehensive review of 20 years of research* (pp. 210-294). Thousand Oaks, CA: Sage.

Kurst-Swanger, K., & Petcosky, J. L. (2003). *Violence in the home: Multidisciplinary perspectives.* New York: Oxford University Press.

Low, S. M., Monarch, N. D., Hartman, S., & Markman, H. (2002). Recent therapeutic advances in the prevention of domestic violence. In P. A. Schewe (Ed.), *Preventing violence in relationships: Interventions across the life span* (pp. 197-217). Washington, DC: American Psychological Association.

Rennison, C. M., & Welchans, S. (2000). *Intimate partner violence.* Washington, DC: Bureau of Justice Statistics. (Publication No. NCJ 178247).

Schewe, P. A. (2002).Conclusion: Past, present, and future directions for preventing violence in relationships. In P. A. Schewe (Ed.), *Preventing violence in relationships: Interventions across the life span* (pp. 263-265). Washington, DC: American Psychological Association

Stith, S. M., Smith, D. B., Penn, C. E., Ward, D. B., & Tritt, D. (2004). Intimate partner physical abuse perpetration and victimization risk factors: A meta-analytic review. *Aggression and Violent Behavior: A Review Journal,* 10, 65-98.

doi:10.1300/J146v13n03_01

CHANGING THE WAY PEOPLE THINK ABOUT INTIMATE PARTNER VIOLENCE

Changing Public Attitudes as a Prevention Strategy to Reduce Intimate Partner Violence

Jacquelyn C. Campbell
Jennifer Manganello

SUMMARY. Although violence by intimate partners has decreased in the past decade, it is still a problem affecting many women. For instance, IPV accounted for 22% of violent crimes against women between 1993 and 1998 (NCVS). The paucity of research evaluating the effectiveness of primary prevention strategies to reduce IPV has been recognized in various reports on intimate partner violence. Experts have suggested that public awareness campaigns would be helpful both to inform abused women about strategies for getting help, and to potentially change pub-

Address correspondence to Jacquelyn C. Campbell, PhD, RN, Johns Hopkins University, School of Nursing, 525 North Wolfe Street, Room 436, Baltimore, MD 21205.

[Haworth co-indexing entry note]: "Changing Public Attitudes as a Prevention Strategy to Reduce Intimate Partner Violence." Campbell, Jacquelyn C., and Jennifer Manganello. Co-published simultaneously in *Journal of Aggression, Maltreatment & Trauma* (The Haworth Maltreatment & Trauma Press, an imprint of The Haworth Press, Inc.) Vol. 13, No. 3/4, 2006, pp. 13-39; and: *Prevention of Intimate Partner Violence* (ed: Sandra M. Stith) The Haworth Maltreatment & Trauma Press, an imprint of The Haworth Press, Inc., 2006, pp. 13-39. Single or multiple copies of this article are available for a fee from The Haworth Document Delivery Service [1-800-HAWORTH, 9:00 a.m. - 5:00 p.m. (EST). E-mail address: docdelivery@haworthpress.com].

lic attitudes and norms about IPV. This article reviews published research available on public education campaigns regarding intimate partner violence, as well as education campaigns conducted for other issues, in order to better understand the potential for success and the limitations of this type of intervention. doi:10.1300/J146v13n03_02 *[Article copies available for a fee from The Haworth Document Delivery Service: 1-800-HAWORTH. E-mail address: <docdelivery@haworthpress.com> Website: <http://www.HaworthPress.com> © 2006 by The Haworth Press, Inc. All rights reserved.]*

KEYWORDS. Intimate partner violence, health education, mass media, prevention, attitudes and norms

The Centers for Disease Control and Prevention (CDC) definition for intimate partner violence (IPV) is used in this article and is summarized as follows: physical and/or sexual violence (use of physical force) or threat of such violence; or psychological/emotional abuse and/or coercive tactics when there has been prior physical and/or sexual violence; between persons who are spouses or non-marital partners (dating, boyfriend-girlfriend) or former spouses or non-marital partners (Saltzman, Fanslow, McMahon, & Shelley, 1999).

Although such violence by intimates has decreased in the past decade, numbers remaining are substantial. In 1998, approximately 900,000 U.S. women reported physical or sexual assault by intimates, reduced from 1.1 million in 1993 (Rennison, 2000). IPV accounted for 22% of violent crimes against women between 1993 and 1998 (vs. 3% for men; Rennison, 2000). Current rates of IPV (in the past year) range from 1.8% to 14% in population-based studies and up to 44% in health care settings (Jones et al., 1999; Tjaden & Thoennes, 2000; Wilt & Olson, 1996). Lifetime estimates vary from 5% to 51% (Bauer, Rodriguez, & Perez-Stable, 2000; Tjaden & Thoennes, 2000), with the most usual range between 25-35%. Women are significantly more likely to be physically or sexually assaulted by a current or former intimate partner than an acquaintance, family member, friend, or stranger (Tjaden & Thoennes, 2000). As high as these figures are, it is commonly accepted that they (particularly crime data) represent underestimates of the true incidence and prevalence of IPV.

The paucity of research evaluating the effectiveness of prevention strategies to reduce IPV, especially primary prevention, has been recognized in various national policy reports on intimate partner violence (Chalk & King, 1998; Cohen, Salmon, & Stobo, 2002; Crowell & Burgess, 1996; U.S. Department of Defense Task Force on Domestic Violence, 2001, 2002). Primary prevention of IPV can be defined as preventing violence between intimate partners before it ever occurs, using strategies that target the entire population or segments at particular risk. One of the most important prevention strategies to reduce conditions that threaten the life and health of large numbers of Americans, therefore recognized as important public health problems, is public awareness or health education campaigns aimed at the entire population or large aggregate groups (e.g., adolescents, a particular ethnic group, or military populations). Experts in the field of IPV have suggested that public awareness campaigns would be helpful both to inform abused women about strategies for getting help and staying safe, and to help change public attitudes and norms about intimate partner violence (e.g., Crowell & Burgess, 1996; Hamby, 1998; Wolfe & Jaffe, 1999).

This article reviews published research available on public education campaigns regarding intimate partner violence in order to better understand the potential for success and the limitations of this type of intervention, with an eventual goal of directing effective public education campaigns to reduce intimate partner violence.

PUBLIC EDUCATION CAMPAIGNS BACKGROUND

Education campaigns are a tool used for political as well as for public health reasons. As Janet Weiss and Mary Tschirhart (1994) state, "public information campaigns are one way that government officials deliberately attempt to shape public attitudes, values, or behavior in the hope of reaching some desirable social outcome" (p. 82). The main assumption of mass media campaigns is that if a message is given to people, they will either change their behavior based on new knowledge, or the message will promote a change in attitudes about an issue, which will lead to a change in behavior (Bettinghaus, 1986).

Education campaigns that use mass media generally include the use of television, radio, newspapers and magazines, and billboards (Bettinghaus, 1986). Weiss and Tschirhart (1994) reviewed over 100 campaigns (government-sponsored in all fields, not just health care) and developed steps to successful campaigns based on the findings. These are: (a) "capture the attention of the right audience," (b) "Deliver a credible message that audiences understand," (c) "Deliver a message that influences the audience," and (d) "Create social contexts that lead toward desired outcomes" (Weiss & Tschirhart, 1994, p. 90).

A variety of theories are used to support and define education campaigns and a few seem to be most relevant with respect to public education campaigns. Although this paper is not intended to provide an in-depth discussion of the theoretical background of education campaigns, it is important to mention theories that are commonly used in order to understand the basis for such campaigns. A more complete listing and description of theories can be found on the Johns Hopkins Center for Communications Programs (JHUCCP) website and also in Piotrow and colleagues (JHUCCP, 2001; Piotrow, Kincaid, Rimon, & Rinehart, 1997). In addition, there is an excellent discussion of theory and communication programs, as well as the application of theory to IPV prevention, in the article in this collection by Ricardo Wray (Wray, this volume). We will briefly describe a few of the most common theories that have been used in developing education campaigns below.

The Theory of Reasoned Action is one theory that has been applied to education campaigns (Atkin, 2001; Kelly, Swaim, & Wayman, 1996; Piotrow et al., 1997). This theory was developed by Martin Fishbein and Icek Azjen. It asserts that people must have an intention to change their behavior to take action, and that intentions are based on attitudes, beliefs, and perceived social norms. The theory suggests that a person's attitude about a behavior is a good prediction of whether or not they will engage in a particular behavior (Cappella, Fishbein, Hornik, Ahern, & Sayeed, 2001; JHUCCP, 2001; Montano & Kasprzyk, 2002; Piotrow et al., 1997). Thus, campaigns designed to influence attitudes and beliefs about behaviors may be informed by this theory.

Another theory relevant to education campaigns is that of social learning, also known as Social Cognitive Theory (Bandura, 2002; Baranowski, Perry, & Parcel, 2002; Cappella et al., 2001; Dignan, Michielutte, Wells, & Bahnson, 1994; JHUCCP, 2001; Marcus, Owen, Forsyth, Cavill, & Fridinger, 1998; Piotrow et al., 1997). The theory identifies several factors that may influence a person's decision to adopt a behavior. For instance, when people believe they are able to or have the skills to make the change (self-efficacy), they are more likely to adopt a behavior. Reinforcement for the behavior and experience that has shown that benefits of the new behavior are greater than the costs may influence behavior change as well (Baranowski et al. 2002; Cappella et al., 2001). This model also implies that people are more likely to change behavior when the desired behavior is modeled, especially by persons with whom identification is possible. For instance,

Piotrow and colleagues (1997) suggest that influential and attractive figures in the media can influence people to engage in behavior change.

The Health Belief Model is also linked to public education campaigns (Atkin, 2001; Cappella et al., 2001; Janz, Champion, & Strecher, 2002). This model relies on how strongly people feel that they are at risk from the issue or behavior being addressed. It also indicates that when people do feel at risk, their belief that the benefits of making changes are greater than the costs, influences their decision to adopt a behavior (Cappella et al., 2001; Janz et al., 2002).

Another theory that could also be used is the stages of change theory, also known as the Transtheoretical Model (JHUCCP, 2001; Marcus et al., 1998; Prochaska, Redding, & Evers, 2002). This theory describes how people go through various stages as they decide whether or not they will adopt a particular behavior. These changes include: precontemplation, contemplation, preparation, action, and maintenance (Prochaska et al., 2002). Media campaigns can help influence this process by tailoring messages that are matched with the readiness for change level of the target population (Marcus et al., 1998).

While these theories are clearly described in the literature on public education campaigns and behavior change, most public education campaigns reviewed in this chapter failed to define what theory they were using in the design and implementation of the campaign. Education campaigns are used to help change public norms and behavior in many areas. However, we know little about how this type of intervention be applied to the field of intimate partner violence and which of the theories used in public education are most applicable to IPV. We review the scant literature on this topic below.

PUBLIC AWARENESS/HEALTH EDUCATION CAMPAIGNS AND INTIMATE PARTNER VIOLENCE: REVIEW OF THE LITERATURE

There is a general consensus that there is a "lack of attention to attitudes and community norms" related to IPV (Fawcett, Heise, Isita-Espejel, & Pick, 1999, p. 41; also Gadomski, Tripp, Wolff, Lewis, & Jenkins, 2001; Woodruff, 1996). In the reviews by both Gadmoski and colleagues (2001) and Wolfe and Jaffe (1999), the only public education campaign discussed is the one conducted by the Advertising Council/Family Violence Prevention Fund.

There has recently been a large increase in published research on IPV interventions in the health care (see Hamberger & Phelan, this volume), law enforcement, and criminal justice systems. There are also beginning to be a few published evaluations of IPV prevention programs that address populations at risk, such as evaluations of dating violence prevention programs (e.g., Foshee, Bauman, Arriaga, Helms, Koch, & Linder, 1998; O'Leary, Woodin, & Timmons, this volume; Wolfe, Werkele, & Scott, 1996) and intervention programs for child witnesses to violence. Yet, there are very few studies that even address interventions aimed to influence public perceptions about the issue or interventions using public education.

There are even fewer articles reporting research related to public education campaigns. Gadomski and colleagues' (2001) article is one of the few that provides an evaluation of an education campaign. The campaign was conducted in a rural area of New York to complement a training program for health care providers about issues related to domestic violence. The training program was completed during the first year of the project, and the media campaign was started during the second year and ran for 7 months (October 1998 to April 1999). The campaign purpose was to increase "public awareness, attitudes and active disapproval as well as to reinforce health provider practice in domestic violence management" by using messages about recognizing IPV and suggesting actions to take when IPV is identified (Gadmoski et al., 2001, p. 268). The target audience was "potential victims and bystanders," not abusers (p. 268). The campaign consisted of radio advertisements, print advertisements, newspaper articles, public speaking events, and posters on bulletin boards.

In order to measure the effect of the campaign, a comparison county (not exposed to the campaign) was selected to match the intervention county based on various health indicators. Telephone interviews were conducted before and after the campaign in both counties using a random digit-dialing representative sample of men and women age 18 to 50. Questions were asked about knowledge, attitudes, and practices relating to domestic violence.

The survey conducted at baseline had an overall response rate of 73% ($n = 240$ intervention group and $n = 138$ control group). The survey conducted after the campaign had a 65% response rate ($n = 433$ intervention group and $n = 200$ control group). In comparing the intervention and comparison responses after the campaign, more intervention than control group respondents reported hearing the campaign slogan (74% vs. 68%) and more intervention group respondents reported hearing or seeing information about domestic violence than those in the control group (83% vs. 77%; p = .03). With respect to how one would respond to an incident of IPV, there was a greater increase in the number of intervention group respondents who were more likely to agree they would talk to the victim (8% intervention vs. 3% control, p = .04). Only responses for one of the six knowledge, attitudes, and practices questions were different before and after the campaign. The intervention group was significantly less likely to agree with the statement "In cases of domestic abuse it is better to leave people alone to work it out themselves than it is to get involved" after the campaign (22% vs. 13%) compared to the control group (33% vs. 14%), although the changes were greater for the control respondents (p = .0008 for comparing changes pre- and post-campaign between the intervention and control groups) (Gadomski et al., 2001).

One other measure of effect was a comparison of calls to the hotline in the intervention county. The number of calls almost doubled from the baseline year to the post-campaign year (520 in 1997 [pre-campaign] vs. 1,145 in 1999 [post-campaign]). Number of calls was not available for the control community. Also, when examining differences between men and women, there were greater changes among men (p = .01) than women in the intervention group before and after the campaign with respect to recognition of the campaign slogan (men 53% vs. 71%; women 77% vs. 77%; p = .004) (Gadomski et al., 2001).

Another study provides an example of how one can use formative research to identify the attitudes of a community and then use this information to develop a communication campaign to try to change those attitudes. Although this study was conducted outside of the United States, it is included in this review due to its unique contribution to the discussion. The researchers used "formative research that included participant observation, eight focus groups with a total of 45 people recruited from the community in question, and five in-depth interviews with abused women" (Fawcett et al., 1999, p. 42). Questions were asked about several issues, including responsibility for this form of violence and strategies to obtain help. Findings suggested that participants believed that issues such as unemployment or problems at work, alcoholism, and financial problems were explanations for violence against women. Also, both men and women seemed to believe that women were somewhat responsible for the violence and that there were reasons for the abuse that were outside of the men's control (they were not fully responsible for their actions; Fawcett et al., 1999).

The results of the formative research led to the development of a campaign that included a workshop for women and a media campaign within the community that used events, posters, and other types of publicity. The campaign message targeted those who were experiencing abuse but had not yet disclosed abuse to anyone. For this reason, the campaign messages included "It's Not Your Fault" for targeting abused women and "The Peacemaker Gains A Lot" for people in the community to encourage getting involved (Fawcett et al., 1999). The communication campaign was still being conducted at the time of publication so no findings regarding success of the campaign have been published.

A similar type of study was conducted in the United States and was targeted at an Arab-American population in a city located in the Midwest (Kulwicki & Miller, 1999). In order to develop an education campaign that would be relevant for Arab-American women, an in-home interview was completed with a convenience sample of 202 women who were clients at an Arab community center in the area. Questions were asked from the Patriarchal Beliefs Questionnaire as well as questions about demographics and beliefs and behaviors about intimate partner violence. The findings were then used to develop an intervention to help change attitudes about IPV. The program involved a media campaign with radio announcements and television shows, community workshops, and distribution of written materials (Kulwicki & Miller, 1999). Post-campaign interviews were not conducted to assess changes in attitudes. Instead, the authors used as evaluation the fact that no women had ever been identified as experiencing IPV at the community center health clinic prior to the campaign, but after the campaign, 70 clients had been identified and referred for services (Kulwicki & Miller, 1999). The authors pointed to a need for more services to accommodate the larger number of women coming forward to obtain help.

"It's Your Business" Campaign

Another recent ethnic group specific media campaign was the "It's Your Business" radio campaign directed to African American listeners and designed by the Family Violence Prevention Fund. This innovative public education campaign used a soap opera or "social drama" type format that has been used extensively in developing countries for various public service campaigns because of the potential for engaging listeners, working from identification with characters that model the looked for behaviors, and stimulating listeners to talk about the topic with others (Wray, Hornik, Gandy, Stryker, Ghez, & Mitchell-Clark, 2002). The campaign was planned to be 12 weeks of 90-second segments and a new segment each week to be aired several times per week during a popular Afrocentric morning rush hour program. Of the four cities that originally committed to the project, only one city aired the program anywhere near the intended rate, and even there the program was shifted from one radio station to another part way through the series. Partly because of this shift, exposure was extremely low (9%) even in that city; however, the measurement of exposure was stringent and well done. Because many people will claim to have heard any public education campaign even before it is aired, in this evaluation only persons who not only claimed to have heard the campaign but also could answer a simple recall question about the storyline and said they had listened to 3 or more episodes were categorized as definitely (moderately) exposed.

The evaluation component in the one city where there was at least some "treatment fidelity" was based on five waves of a random sample telephone survey with a sample size of 385 pre-campaign and 698 post-campaign. Those exposed to the campaign demonstrated positive changes in attitude in 21 of the 27 items, with 10 of the 27 showing a significant difference; low power related to the low exposure rate decreased the chances of finding significance (Wray et al., 2002). Additional discussion of this campaign, including the theoretical approach used to inform the campaign and lessons learned, can be found in Wray (this issue).

Family Violence Prevention Fund "There's No Excuse" Campaign

The most detailed research to date regarding a public education campaign and its relationship to public awareness, attitudes, and intimate partner violence is discussed in *Ending Domestic Violence* (Klein, Campbell, Soler, & Ghez, 1997). The Family Violence Prevention Fund (FVPF) used a combination of lessons learned in many years of addressing IPV (pre-campaign survey and focus group data, lessons from other fields, and advice from public relations specialists) to design a public service campaign to change public attitudes about domestic violence. It was noted that although the majority of people in the United States agree that IPV is wrong, they "demonstrate covert attitudes which implicitly condone battering, and which create an environment in which inaction is the norm rather than the exception" (Ghez, 1995, p. 2). For example, the 1992 EDK Associates pre-campaign poll found that although 83% of Americans would say something disapproving to a friend if he said he had slapped his wife, this was a significantly lower percentage compared to people who said they would insist on driving a drunk friend home (95%) (Klein et al., 1997). From the review of successful campaigns about other issues (recycling, smoking, colon cancer awareness, and drinking and driving), the following shared attributes were found: the use of "simple, powerful messages," targeted use of the media, knowledge about the target audience, using messages that people can relate to, highlighting positive outcomes of behavior change, use of well-known spokespeople, and continued efforts as opposed to a short-term project (Ghez, 1995, p. 3). Twelve ethnic and gender specific focus groups were conducted in five cities in order to help shape the message in the campaign. The television, print, and bumper sticker "There's No Excuse" campaign resulted from this work and was distributed nationwide in 1994-95. The book *Ending Domestic Violence* (Klein et al., 1997) reports the data from the original EDK poll ($N = 1600$, including an ethnic specific survey of 300 African American and 300 Latino participants) and focus groups as well as the campaign evaluation data conducted by Lieberman Research Incorporated. The Lieberman polls included a baseline or benchmark national random survey conducted just before the campaign in 1994 and two rounds of post campaign polling in 1995 ($N = 700+$ each). All surveys were population based telephone surveys, but unfortunately, the Lieberman surveys did not over sample in ethnic minority groups and therefore resulted in cell sizes too small to analyze ethnic groups separately. The Lieberman polls were also less extensive than the original EDK survey, although several of the elements were the same or comparable.

The polls had other limitations, namely not being designed by researchers, not utilizing comparison groups, and primarily descriptive statistics used in the overall analysis (Klein et al., 1997). Nonetheless, the sampling techniques were sound, and the data is useful in at least suggesting the effectiveness of the campaign. There were significant positive changes in concern about IPV and willingness to take action between 1992 and 1994 that the investigators attributed to the widespread publicity about the domestic violence aspects of the O.J. Simpson case during that time period. Men's attitudes seemed to be most affected by the 1994 campaign, with an increase from 25% to 33% indicating that they thought domestic violence (DV) was a serious problem (compared to 44% of women both before and after the campaign). The other demographic group demonstrating the most change was city dwellers. Similarly, significantly more Americans overall said that DV was extremely or very important after the campaign, with the most change amongst men and city dwellers but also an increase among suburban dwellers, who nonetheless remained less concerned than city or rural residents. Significantly more of the respondents (29% to 35%) reported knowing a woman who was physically abused, especially among the relatively young (18-34), city dwellers, and those of middle income ($20-39,000 per year) in contrast to those of below or above that range in income. Although the proportion of respondents saying that DV needs outside intervention was extremely high both before and after the campaign if there was physical violence resulting in injuries needing medical attention (97-99%), the proportion saying such hitting without injury needed outside intervention increased from 80% to 87%, with a similar increase in those saying shouting curses and pounding on a table (19% to 28%) was not just a private matter. The gains in the last two areas decreased as the campaign wound down (to 82% and 24%, respectively) but not to pre-campaign levels.

Attitude change does not always result in behavior change. Perhaps the most encouraging results in the polling were in terms of reported action in regards to IPV (Klein et al., 1997). Eighteen percent of respondents said they had taken action against domestic violence (ranging from donating money to calling the police to intervening in a fight) in the year before the campaign (in comparison to 56% and 43% taking action in regards to the environment and poor children, respectively), while 21% said they had immediately after the campaign and 24% 10 months later. The largest increase was in talking to an abused woman, increasing from 9% pre-campaign to 16% and 17% in the polls after the campaign. The groups who increased their participation the most were those who knew an abused woman, those 18-34, city dwellers, and those in the lowest income group (< $20,000). Although these proportions are low, when other possible actions were suggested to participants in the last poll, between 54% and 70% of participants said they would be willing to do at least one of the suggested actions. Across all of the data reported, men were less impressed with the importance of DV than women, and women took more action to begin with and changed more in their actions than did men. In the original EDK polling, men in each ethnic group lagged behind women in that ethnic group in both attitudes and behavior about DV.

The "Soul City" Initiative and Evaluation

"Soul City" was an innovative project implemented in South Africa in 1999 that consisted of a 13-part prime time serialized TV drama, a 45-part radio drama in 9 languages, and 1 million each of three information booklets. The campaign purpose was to disseminate information on how to prevent domestic violence, sexual harassment, HIV, and hypertension. The campaign also gave information on small business establishment and personal finance management. An innovative partnership of Non Governmental Organizations (NGOs) funded and designed the project, with the evaluation component funded by the European Union. The DV content expert NGO partner was the National Network for Violence Against Women (NNVAW), the major DV advocacy organization in South Africa.

The independent evaluation component of "Soul City" used theoretical, methodological, and researcher triangulation and was based first on surveys administered to a national random sample of households (with rural areas less well sampled), with in-person interviews by a large group of trained field workers in the language of the participant's choice (Institute for Health and Development Communication, 2001). There were 2,000 interviews pre-campaign and another 2,000 post-campaign. In addition, there was a cost analysis and a sentinel site (1 urban and 1 rural) component of the evaluation consisting of a longitudinal panel design with 4 waves of survey ($N = 829$ Black South Africans, with approximately 18% attrition), 97 in-depth interviews of a subset of participants who shifted in attitude and a subsample of those that did not, local media monitoring, collection of existing data from related organizations, and a community mobilization component including interviews of community leaders and other key informants. At least three notable limitations in the survey component of the evaluation were the lack of appropriate training regarding referral and advocacy for DV, a less random sample from rural areas, and some bias in the female DV attitudes section depending on whether males versus females interviewed women. However, the evaluation had many strengths including the gender matching analysis, the multimodal evaluation components, triangulation, and several strategic sampling strategies.

An excellent media saturation was achieved with good exposure rates of 79% of the target population for the TV and/or radio programming (Institute for Health and Development Communication, 2001). The evaluation design was in terms of relative exposure, with no pamphlet, radio and/or TV types of exposure. In terms of DV outcomes, there were significant changes in attitudes and intentions to confront abusers, refer victims, report DV, and talk to victims about DV (OR = 6.4). Other outcomes with significant differences according to levels of exposure were recall of hearing hotline information (16, 37, 45, 61%), and the behaviors of writing down the hotline number (0, 12, 15, 25%), doing something about DV (9, 12, 14, 16%) and talking to someone (e.g., friends, family, co-workers) about DV (17, 36, 39, 51%). Approximately 8% of respondents said they were current victims of intimate partner violence, and there was a significant difference according to level of exposure in actually making hotline calls (1, 2, 4, 5%). In an innovative part of the evaluation, community action was also measured both through the in-depth interviews with many reporting "bottle or pot banging" when they observed domestic violence, including psychological abuse, in public, as had been suggested in the campaign. Public protest against DV was also measured as an outcome, with 1% reporting such protest if no exposure to "Soul City" and 3.3% and 5% as the levels of exposure increased. The evaluation team also felt that the first South African law addressing domestic violence (the Domestic Violence Act of 1999) was passed, in part because of the publicity and public support generated from the "Soul City" initiative.

Child Abuse Media Campaigns

Since there are so few published research reports available regarding violence between partners and education campaign evaluation, two additional articles are included in this review that focus on the child abuse educational campaigns. One article discusses various community-level interventions for preventing child abuse (Hay & Jones, 1994). The authors suggest that public education campaigns and media messages designed to prevent child abuse (with different messages designed for different target groups) can be a useful strategy, and that the ways media portrays families can influence social norms and attitudes as well (Hay & Jones, 1994).

Another research team actually evaluated a media campaign designed to increase public action to help abused children in families with substance abuse problems (Andrews, McLeese, & Curran, 1995). The campaign was based on the theory of social action, which suggests that people are more likely to perform an activity when they believe their action will have a specific outcome. Conducted in South Carolina, "the project was designed to increase statewide public awareness of the association between child maltreatment and alcohol and other drug abuse, promote access to services for families affected by both problems, and strengthen collaboration among child welfare and addictions professionals" (Andrews et al., 1995, p. 923).

Focus groups and telephone surveys were completed first in order to help develop campaign messages. The campaign then utilized television, billboards, posters, and print publications in order to encourage people to call a toll-free number if they or someone they knew needed help (Andrews et al., 1995, p. 928). A survey conducted halfway through the campaign found that 61% of respondents reported exposure to the campaign message (with 88.8% of those reporting exposure through television) (Andrews et al., 1995). The number of calls made to the phone number also showed that the campaign had an effect, as the number of calls increased as the campaign spread and continued to increase over time (Andrews et al., 1995).

Other Media Coverage of Domestic Violence

It is important to mention that one of the implications of the growing attention given to the issue of family violence is that it receives more widespread exposure in the media, especially in the news but also in entertainment shows. As previously mentioned, Klein and colleagues (1997) hypothesized that the changes in increased awareness and increased ranking of importance of domestic violence between their first two polls was related to the news coverage of the O.J. Simpson trial. Yet, this type of coverage has not been studied in detail. As Mia Consalvo said in her paper that reviewed the portrayal of domestic violence in the television series *Cops*, "media attention to the issue of domestic violence in both news and entertainment has increased, but with unknown results. Very little scholarly work has looked at media depictions and coverage of domestic violence. What then, are the accounts 'saying'? Who is doing the telling? What is the underlying message being conveyed?" (Consalvo, 1998, p. 1). Also, it is not clear how coverage of domestic violence influences people who are exposed to the coverage.

Studies have tried to improve the understanding of how the media reflects social norms regarding domestic violence and how the portrayal of domestic violence has changed over time. Studies have also examined how the news frames domestic violence. There have been sociological studies that have examined the portrayal of domestic violence in the news, women's magazines, reality television, literature, and movies. Such studies have been informative and useful with respect to understanding how the media reflects social norms regarding domestic violence, and how the portrayal of domestic violence has changed over time. There have also been studies specifically related to reporting of domestic violence in the news.

One researcher, Meyers (1997), conducted a study employing both content analysis and interviews to examine the portrayal of domestic violence in the news. Her book *News Coverage of Violence Against Women* mostly examined the portrayal of female victims of crime in the news, discussing issues such as 'blaming the victim,' 'good girl/bad girl' representations, and how journalists cover crime news. Another author, Cuklanz (1996), explored media coverage of rape trials in her book *Rape on Trial*. She discussed several cases and how they were represented in the media, and examined thematic vs. episodic coverage, finding a greater portrayal of events versus themes (Cuklanz, 1996). Another study compared coverage of domestic violence in three major newspapers before and after the O.J. Simpson case to determine whether any changes in the frequency and nature of coverage could be observed. The researchers expected that there would be a greater number of articles about domestic violence, and that there would be fewer incident articles and greater coverage of domestic violence as an issue (Maxwell, Huxford, Borum, & Hornik, 2000). The results indicated that although the frequency of coverage increased, the content did not experience any significant changes (Maxwell et al., 2000).

Media Advocacy Campaigns

As contrasted with education campaigns to try to directly influence individual attitudes and behavior, media advocacy is used to attempt to change policy with the idea that policy change can eventually influence both attitudes and behavior concerning various health issues. Wallack and Dorfman (1996) identified three main functions of media advocacy, including agenda setting (getting the issue on the public agenda), framing of an issue (getting the issue presented by the media in a certain way), and the advancement of policies designed to provide solutions to issues. They also suggest that this type of intervention can be more effective for changing behavior than campaigns aimed at influencing individuals (Wallack & Dorfman, 2001). Further discussion of media advocacy can be found in Wray (this volume).

One of the only published studies related to media advocacy and domestic violence was targeted at efforts to reduce sexist alcohol advertisements that can potentially increase violence against women (Woodruff, 1996). An effort called the "Dangerous Promises Campaign" began in three California cities to alter how alcohol advertisers portrayed women in their ads. After communicating directly with various industry associations, and getting little positive response, the coalition chose to advance their goals using media advocacy. The group also attempted to use billboards and to shape the framing of news stories related to their efforts. In the end, although the group achieved some successes, Woodruff indicated that other advocacy activities are necessary as well, and that it takes a great deal of time and effort to maintain press coverage over a long-term period. This study did not examine any changes in public attitudes that may have occurred as a result of this campaign.

PUBLIC AWARENESS/HEALTH EDUCATION CAMPAIGNS: LESSONS LEARNED FROM OTHER FIELDS

Although the research concerning education campaigns and intimate partner violence is fairly limited, there are studies in other health-related areas that have direct implications for developing media campaigns to prevent interpersonal violence. A summary of research related to the effectiveness of anti-smoking campaigns, substance abuse, and youth violence prevention efforts, as well as from general health-related campaigns will be presented next.

Anti-Smoking Campaigns

One of the most common health issues discussed in the literature is tobacco control and the movement to reduce smoking. For example, Brian Flay (1987) examined 40 different campaigns that had been conducted prior to 1986. These campaigns varied in their messages, but some of the more common ones were providing information about negative health effects, offering reasons and motivation to quit smoking, and providing details about where to get help to quit. Flay describes successes and limitations of the different types of campaigns, and in the end, concludes that while it seems that the media can be influential in influencing attitudes and behavior about smoking, programs vary a great deal in their effectiveness. In his conclusions, he states, "the very best programs were much more effective than the worst or even the average, yet the published reports provide very few ideas on why some were more successful and others less so" (Flay, 1987, p. 158).

Erickson, McKenna, and Romano (1990), in their review of media campaigns with respect to smoking from the 1950s though the 1980s, highlighted both strengths and limitations of the media's ability to influence smoking behaviors. They suggest that while media campaigns can "increase knowledge, change attitudes, reinforce attitudes, provide cues to simple action, and demonstrate simple skills" (Erickson et al., 1990, p. 240), they are limited by the fact that media can only influence those who are exposed to it, and conclude that media alone is generally not successful in getting people to stop smoking.

More recent studies (Jenkins, McPhee, Le, Pham, Ha, & Stewart, 1997; Sly, Hopkins, Trapido, & Ray, 2001) conclude that although earlier studies found inconclusive evidence regarding the media campaigns and a change in smoking attitudes and behaviors, more recent studies have begun to show positive findings. For example, one of the largest anti-smoking campaigns discussed in the literature, the "Tobacco Education Media Campaign," conducted in California from 1990 to 1991, reported that as a result of the campaign, youth demonstrated changes in attitudes in the desired direction, with greater numbers of smokers thinking of quitting and fewer non-smoking youths thinking about starting to smoke. Also, exposed youths were significantly more likely to report greater changes in attitudes than unexposed youths ($p <$ .0025; Popham, Potter, Hetrick, Muthen, Duerr, & Johnson, 1994).

Two studies designed to reduce or prevent smoking targeted specific ethnic groups. Jenkins et al. (1997) targeted men of Vietnamese-American descent in the San Francisco area and Boyd et al. (1998) targeted African Americans. Jenkins and colleagues reported that the campaign, which included newspaper and television advertisements, distribution of educational materials, and billboards, "produced both a significant decrease in smoking prevalence and a significant increase in quitting among men in the intervention community relative to men in the comparison community" (p. 1033). The authors attributed the successes of this campaign to the length of campaign time (2 years), the additional part of the intervention that targeted students and families, and the fact that messages were reinforced by a statewide campaign (Jenkins et al., 1997). However, while Boyd et al. (1998), in their discussion of the campaign that utilized radio and television advertisements as well as outreach efforts to increase the number of African Americans calling a Cancer Information Service help line for information about how to quit smoking, reported that while the number of calls was greater in the intervention compared to the control areas ($p <$ .008), calls returned to baseline rates within approximately four weeks of the campaign.

Substance Abuse Campaigns

A number of campaigns have been focused on raising awareness about alcohol use and influencing attitudes about drunk driving. Yanovitzky and Bennett (1999), after reviewing the literature on this topic, conclude that only campaigns implementing enforcement programs in addition to media campaigns showed any measurable effect, but point out that even then such effects were mostly short-term. Likewise, DeJong and Wallack (1999), in their discussion of the Office of National Drug Control Policy's media campaign in 1998, reported that campaigns designed only to generate awareness about a problem are often not successful, and that interventions require additional components to actually result in behavior change. Similarly, studies related to drug use prevention and media campaigns found little evidence of successful outcomes due to "unrealistic objectives or lack of specific objectives, short-run efforts, failure to communicate benefits to viewers and lack of market segmentation" (Bandy & President, 1983, pp. 266-67). In a more recent evaluation of a campaign targeting substance abuse, the authors suggest that media campaigns that are conducted for a short time or are national as opposed to being targeted to specific communities are less likely to be successful (Kelly et al., 1996).

Health Oriented Campaigns

Cancer screening is another area that has utilized public education campaigns to increase knowledge about prevention techniques such as screening. Dignan et al. (1994) focused on raising awareness about cervical cancer screening and targeted Black women in an area of North Carolina, and Jenkins, McPhee, Bird, Pham, Nguyen, and Nguyen (1999) focused on raising awareness about both breast and cervical cancer screening in Vietnamese-American communities. While both studies reported increases in awareness, both also report limited success with increasing screening rates for women. Jenkins et al. (1999) suggest that possible reasons for the limited success are that the length of the campaign was too short and that there was no program specifically targeting health providers.

Education campaigns have also been applied to issues of nutrition and healthy eating. The "1% Or Less" campaign was conducted for six weeks in a community in West Virginia (Reger, Wootan, & Booth-Butterfield, 1999). It used both paid advertisements and public events to try to increase the use of low-fat milk. Another community with similar characteristics was selected as the comparison group. When comparing milk sales at different grocery stores before and after the campaign, sales of low-fat milk increased in the intervention community but not in the control community and these differences remained after six months. In addition, pre- and post-campaign telephone surveys in each community showed similar results regarding what types of milk were purchased. The authors suggest the success of the "1% Or

Less" campaign was in part due to the use of one message that was directed at a particular behavior and was easy to understand (Reger et al., 1999). They also point out that this success was achieved even without other types of interventions, while many campaigns require the use of non-media efforts to support media efforts (Reger et al., 1997).

Campaigns to increase exercise and physical activity are a related area where education campaigns have been used. Marcus et al. (1998) examined seven studies that discussed campaigns that focused on messages related to reducing risk factors for cardiovascular disease (CVD) and one that emphasized only physical activity. They found that 70% of respondents across all studies were able to recall the messages of the campaigns (Marcus et al., 1998). Still, there was little evidence of change in knowledge, and inconclusive findings regarding changes in behavior (Marcus et al., 1998).

The most positive findings on the use of public awareness campaigns to influence physical activity came from the Stanford Five-City Project, a "6-year education intervention (1980-1986) targeted all residents in two treatment communities and involved a multiple risk factor strategy delivered through multiple educational methods" (Fortmann & Varady, 2000, p. 316). Marcus et al. (1998) report that the treatment group of men reported greater amounts of time spent in 'vigorous activities.' Bellicha and McGrath (1990) provide indicate that the study:

> . . . demonstrated that certain risk-reduction behaviors, for example, improved eating habits, could be learned through mass media alone when behavior change depended primarily on acquiring new knowledge. Other risk-reduction behaviors, such as smoking cessation, required mass media supplemented with skills training, face-to-face communication, social support, and other interventions to be successful. (p. 247)

Lessons learned from all of the studies reviewed by Marcus et al. (1998) suggest that developing a campaign that targets a specific population and matching messages to how ready people were to make changes seemed to result in the most substantial changes.

HIV/AIDS Campaigns

HIV/AIDS is another public health issue that has been the target of some educational efforts. Much of the work in this area has been done in other countries and several studies report positive findings (Karlyn, 2001; Myhre & Flora, 2000; Ross, Rigby, Rosser, Anagnostou, & Brown, 1990; Yoder, Hornik, & Chirwa, 1996). In a review article of 41 studies from 17 different countries, Myrhe and Flora (2000) provide four suggestions for HIV/AIDS campaigns based on study findings. These include: (a) "better reporting of media campaign components and outcomes," (b) "more systematic evaluation," (c) "greater integration of theory," and (d) "increased attention to community wide intervention strategies" (p. 29).

Conclusions Drawn from Non-IPV Campaigns

In conclusion, results of media campaigns in changing public health-related behaviors seem to be mixed and positive findings seem to be fairly minimal (Bettinghaus, 1986). In a meta-analysis of 48 campaigns, Snyder et al. (2004) found that "the effects ranged from $r = .07$ to $r = .10$, and in percentage terms, campaigns changed the behavior of about 8% of the population" (p. 89; Snyder, 2001). Furthermore, more people were likely to start new behaviors (12%, $r = .12$) than to stop behaviors (5%, $r = .05$) as a result of exposure to campaigns (Snyder, 2001).

Wallack (1981), citing Lazarsfeld and Merton (1948/1975), offers three requirements that lead to more effective campaigns. These are "monopolization," meaning there are no other counter-messages to oppose the campaign message; "canalization," which suggests that campaigns are more successful when they attempt to alter current behaviors as opposed to trying to encourage a complete shift in behaviors; and "supplementation," meaning additional interventions that involve personal communication should be implemented in addition to mass media educational efforts (Wallack, 1981, pp. 232-234).

Other authors share some of these lessons and present new ones. Many mention the need for better evaluation of campaigns and better definition of outcome variable and measurement of these outcomes (Reger et al., 1999; Wallack, 1984; Wilde, 1993). They suggest that differences in how campaigns are evaluated make it difficult to compare findings (Bettinghaus, 1986). Another common theme is that media campaigns are more successful when combined with other interventions (for instance, laws or personal counseling) (Bettinghaus, 1986; Boyd et al., 1998; Marcus et al., 1998; Snyder, 2001; Wallack, 1984; Yanovitzky & Bennett, 1999). Having a specific target audience also seems to help increase the success of campaigns (Boyd et al., 1998;

Marcus et al., 1998; Gadomski et al., 2001). Establishing clear messages about what the desired behavior would be is important to ensure that a campaign will have the intended effect (Gadomski et al., 2001). In addition, campaigns that continue for longer periods of time seem to be more effective (Bettinghaus, 1986).

CONCLUSIONS

From the few evaluations of media educational campaigns in domestic violence, there is some, albeit meager, support for believing that a well designed and tailored media campaign can indeed change attitudes and perhaps have some effect on behavior. It is somewhat ironic that the most ambitious and best evaluated campaign was conducted in a developing country; the South African "Soul City" project is in many ways the most encouraging, in terms of the innovation of both the campaign itself and the evaluation. In addition to the relatively scant empirical research on the impact of public education campaigns in the field of DV, there is expertise to draw from. When planning an education campaign for issues of IPV, Ghez (1995) recommends having a "clear understanding of what motivates the target audience to get involved in stopping domestic violence," understanding "barriers to intervention," knowing "how the public understands domestic violence" to develop a way to frame the issue that people can accept, and developing different messages that target particular communities (p. 4). Most experts and some empirical research from the EDK ethnic specific focus groups suggest that culture and ethnicity are important in shaping campaigns.

The lack of an agreed upon theory to explain why people engage in intimate partner violence makes it difficult to develop a campaign. Fawcett and colleagues (1999) discuss how it is easier to develop messages for other areas, such as tobacco control and AIDS prevention, as they have better defined theories about the behavior and clearer desired outcomes (for instance, use of a condom). Defining a target population and establishing clear messages about what the desired behavior would be is important to ensure that a campaign will have the intended effect (Gadomski et al., 2001). Other factors that are important when designing an education campaign, as discussed by Gadomski et al., are deciding whether to focus on social norms or individual norms, providing messages that do not further endanger women, and establishing clear messages about what the desired behaviors are (Gadomski et al., 2001). Also from Gadomski et al.'s work one can conclude that a campaign addressed to the general population combined with training for providers is a good strategy and that ensuring services are available is another component that can add to the success of the campaign.

From evaluations in other arenas, such as anti-smoking and HIV/AIDS campaigns, several other important lessons can be learned. Gains are difficult to maintain, so a sustained, long-term approach is necessary. Several studies suggest that the use of non-media efforts (e.g., laws or personal communication) to support media efforts are helpful (e.g., Reger et al., 1999; Wallack, 1984) and in fact may be necessary to actually result in behavior change (DeJong & Wallack, 1999). Developing a campaign that targets a specific population and matching messages to how ready people were to make changes seemed to result in the most substantial changes (e.g., Marcus et al., 1998). In Wallack's (1981) language, "monopolization" (no other counter-messages) and "canalization" (trying to alter current behaviors rather than encouraging a total shift) are also useful (pp. 232-234).

Many authors discuss the need for better evaluation of campaigns and better definition of outcome variable and measurement of these outcomes (Reger et al., 1999; Wallack, 1984; Wilde, 1993). In addition, differences in how campaigns are evaluated make it difficult to compare findings (Bettinghaus, 1986). It is also necessary to have some comparison group in order to really attribute any change to a campaign, a design element missing in most of the evaluations reviewed. Such evaluations can be expensive and funding sources for this kind of research are difficult to secure.

There is great potential for prevention of domestic violence through the use of intelligent, well-designed media educational campaigns coupled with strategic use of press releases and other forms of news media. Yet in order for us to know if these campaigns are effective and what components should be replicated, rigorous, well-designed, and funded evaluations are also necessary.

REFERENCES

Andrews, A. B., McLeese, D. G., & Curran, S. (1995). The impact of a media campaign on public action to help maltreated children in addictive families. *Child Abuse and Neglect, 19*(8), 921-932.

Atkin, C. K. (2001). Theories and principles of media health campaigns. In R. E. Rice & C. K. Atkin (Eds.), *Public communication campaigns* (pp. 49-68). Thousand Oaks, CA: Sage Publications.

Bandura, A. (2002). Social cognitive theory of mass communication. In J. Bryant & D. Zillman (Eds.), *Media effects: Advances in theory and research* (2nd ed., pp. 121-154). Mahwah, NJ: Lawrence Erlbaum Associates.

Bandy, P., & President, P.A. (1983). Recent literature on drug abuse prevention and mass media: Focusing on youth, parents, women and the elderly. *Journal of Drug Education, 13*(3), 255-271.

Baranowski, T., Perry, C.L., & Parcel, G.S. (2002). How individuals, environments, and health behavior interact: Social Cognitive Theory. In K. Glanz, B.K. Rimer, & F.M. Lewis (Eds.), *Health behavior and health education: Theory, research and practice* (3rd ed., pp. 165-184). San Francisco, CA: Jossey-Bass.

Bauer, H. M., Rodriguez, M. A., & Perez-Stable, E. J. (2000). Prevalence and determinants of intimate partner abuse among public hospital primary care patients. *Journal of General Internal Medicine, 15*(11), 811-817.

Bellicha, T., & McGrath, J. (1990). Mass media approaches to reducing cardiovascular risk. *Public Health Reports, 105*(3), 245-252.

Bettinghaus, E. P. (1986). Health promotion and the knowledge-attitude-behavior continuum. *American Journal of Preventive Medicine, 15*(5), 475-491.

Boyd, N. R., Sutton, C., Orleans, C. T., McClatchey, M. W., Bingler, R., Fleisher, L. et al. (1998). Quit today! A targeted communications campaign to increase use of the caner information service by African American Smokers. *Preventive Medicine, 27*(S), 50-60.

Cappella, J. N., Fishbein, M., Hornik, R., Ahern, R. K., & Sayeed, S. (2001). Using theory to select messages in anti-drug media campaigns. In R. E. Rice & C. K. Atkin (Eds.), *Public communication campaigns* (pp. 214-230). Thousand Oaks, CA: Sage Publications.

Chalk, R., & King, P. (Eds.). (1998). *Violence in families: Assessing prevention and treatment programs.* Washington, DC: National Academy Press.

Cohen, F., Salmon, M., & Stobo, J. (2002). *Confronting chronic neglect: The education and training of health professionals on family violence.* Washington, DC: National Academy Press.

Consalvo, M. (1998). Hegemony, domestic violence and 'cops': A critique of concordance. *Journal of Popular Film and Television, Summer 26*(2), 62-70.

Crowell, N. A., & Burgess, A. W. (1996). *Understanding violence against women.* Washington, DC: National Academy Press.

Cuklanz, L. M. (1996). *Rape on trial.* Philadelphia, PA: University of Pennsylvania.

DeJong, W., & Wallack, L. (1999). A critical perspective on the drug Czar's antidrug media campaign. *Journal of Health Communication, 4*(2), 155-60.

Dignan, M., Michielutte, R., Wells, H. B., & Bahnson, J. (1994). The Forsyth-county cervical-cancer prevention project: Cervical-cancer screening for black women. *Health Education Research, 9*(4), 411-420.

Erickson, A. C., McKenna, J. W., & Romano, R. M. (1990). Past lessons and new uses of the mass media in reducing tobacco consumption. *Public Health Report, 105*(3), 239-244.

Fawcett, G., Heise, L., Isita-Espejel, L., & Pick, S. (1999). Changing community responses to wife abuse: A research and demonstration project in Iztacalco, Mexico. *American Psychologist, 54*(1), 41-49.

Flay, B. (1987). Mass media and smoking cessation: A critical review. *American Journal of Public Health, 77*(2), 153-160.

Fortmann, S. P., & Varady, A. N. (2000). Effects of a community-wide health education program on cardiovascular disease morbidity and mortality: The Stanford five-city project. *American Journal of Epidemiology, 152*(4), 316-23.

Foshee, V. A., Bauman, K. E., Arriaga, X. B., Helms, R. W., Koch, G. G., & Linder, G. F. (1998). An evaluation of safe dates, and adolescent dating violence prevention program. *American Journal of Public Health, 88*(1), 45-50.

Gadomski, A., Tripp, M., Wolff, D., Lewis, C., & Jenkins, P. (2001). Impact of a rural domestic violence prevention campaign. *Journal of Rural Health, 17*(3), 266-277.

Ghez, M. (1995). *Communication and public education: Effective tools to promote a cultural change on domestic violence.* Revision of paper presented at the Violence Against Women Strategic Planning Committee, National Institute of Justice, Washington DC. Retrieved April 23, 2001, from http://wwwfvpf.org/publiced/nij.html

Hamberger, L. K., & Phelan, M. B. (2006). Domestic violence screening in medical and mental health care settings: Overcoming barriers to screening, identifying, and helping partner violence victims. *Journal of Aggression, Maltreatment, & Trauma, 13*(3/4), 61-99.

Hamby, S. L. (1998). Partner violence: Prevention and intervention. In J. Jasinski & L. Williams (Eds.), *Partner violence: A comprehensive review of 20 years of research* (pp. 210-258). Thousand Oaks, CA: Sage.

Hay, T., & Jones, L. (1994). Societal interventions to prevent child abuse and neglect. *Child Welfare, 73*(5), 379-403.

Institute for Health and Development Communication. (2001). *Soul City 4: Evaluation methodology, volume 1.* Retrieved from, http://www.soulcity.ac.za

Janz, N. K., Champion, V. L., & Strecher, V. J. (2002). The Health Belief Model. In K. Glanz, B. K. Rimer, & F. M. Lewis (Eds.), *Health behavior and health education: Theory, research and practice* (3rd ed., pp. 45-66). San Francisco, CA: Jossey-Bass.

Jenkins, C. N., McPhee, S. J., Bird, J. A., Pham, G. Q., Nguyen, B. H., & Nguyen, T. (1999). Effect of a media-led education campaign on breast and cervical cancer screening among Vietnamese-American women. *Preventive Medicine, 28*(4), 395-406.

Jenkins, C. N., McPhee, S. J., Le, A., Pham, G. Q., Ha, N. T., & Stewart, S. (1997). The effectiveness of a media-led intervention to reduce smoking among Vietnamese-American men. *American Journal of Public Health, 87*(6), 1031-4.

Johns Hopkins Center for Communication Programs. (2001). *Research and evaluation theoretical framework* [database]. Retrieved December 7, 2001 from http://www.jhuccp.org/r&e/retheory.stm

Jones, A. A., Gielen, A. C., Campbell, J. C., Schollenberger, J., Dienemann, J. A., Kub, J. et al. (1999). Annual and lifetime prevalence of partner abuse in a sample of female HMO enrollees. *Women's Health Issues, 9*(6), 295-305.

Karlyn, A. S. (2001). The impact of a targeted radio campaign to prevent STIs and HIV/AIDS in Mozambique. *AIDS Education and Prevention, 13*(5), 438-451.

Kelly, K. J., Swaim, R. C., & Wayman, J. C. (1996). The impact of a localized anti-drug media campaign on targeted variables associated with adolescent drug use. *Journal of Public Policy and Marketing, 15*(2), 238-251.

Klein, E., Campbell, J. C., Soler, E., & Ghez, M. (1997). *Ending domestic violence: Changing public perceptions/halting the epidemic.* Thousand Oaks, CA: Sage Publications.

Kulwicki, A. D., & Miller, J. (1999). Domestic violence in the Arab American population: Transforming environmental conditions through community education. *Issues in Mental Health Nursing, 20,* 199-215.

Lazarsfeld, P. F., & Merton, R. K. (1948/1975). Mass communication, popular taste and organized social action. Reprinted from *The Communication of Ideas.* New York, Institute for Religious and Social Studies, 1948. In W. Schramm (Ed), *Mass Communications.* Second edition, third printing. Urbana, IL: University of Illinois Press, 1975.

Marcus, B. H., Owen, N., Forsyth, L. H., Cavill, N. A., & Fridinger, F. (1998). Physical activity interventions using mass media, print media, and information technology. *American Journal of Preventive Medicine, 15*(4), 362-378.

Maxwell, K., Huxford, J., Borum, C., & Hornik, R. (2000). Covering domestic violence: How the OJ Simpson case shaped reporting of domestic violence in the news media. *Journalism and Mass Communication Quarterly, 77*(2), 258-272.

Meyers, M. (1997). *New coverage of violence against women.* Newbury Park: Sage Publications.

Montano, D.E., & Kasprzyk, D. (2002). The Theory of Reasoned Action and the Theory of Planned Behavior. In K. Glanz, B.K. Rimer, & F.M. Lewis (Eds.), *Health behavior and health education: Theory, research and practice* (3rd ed., pp. 67-98). San Francisco, CA: Jossey-Bass.

Myhre, S. L., & Flora, J. A. (2000). HIV/AIDS communication campaigns: Progress and prospects. *Journal of Health Communication, 5*(2), 29-45.

O'Leary, K. D., Woodin, E. M., & Fritz, P. A. (2006). Can we prevent the hitting? Recommendations for preventing intimate partner violence between young adults. *Journal of Aggression, Maltreatment & Trauma, 13*(3/4), 121-178.

Piotrow, P. T., Kincaid, D. L., Rimon, J. G., & Rinehart, W. (1997). *Health communication: Lessons from family planning and reproductive health.* Westport, CT: Praeger.

Popham, W. J., Potter, L. D., Hetrick, M. A., Muthen, L. K., Duerr, J. M., & Johnson, M. D. (1994). Effectiveness of the California 1990-1991 tobacco education media campaign. *American Journal of Preventive Medicine, 10*(6), 310-326.

Prochaska, J. O., Redding, C. A., & Evers, K. E. (2002). The Transtheoretical Model and stages of change. In K. Glanz, B. K. Rimer, & F. M. Lewis (Eds.), *Health behavior and health education: Theory, research and practice* (3rd ed., pp. 99-120). San Francisco, CA: Jossey-Bass.

Reger, B., Wootan, M. G., & Booth-Butterfield, S. (1999). Using mass media to promote healthy eating: A community-based demonstration project. *Preventive Medicine, 29*(5), 414-421.

Rennison, C. M. (2000). *Criminal victimization 1999: Changes 1998-99 with trends 1993-99.* Washington DC: US Department of Justice, Bureau of Justice Statistics (NCJ 182734).

Ross, M. W., Rigby, K., Rosser, B. R. S., Anagnostou, P., & Brown, M. (1990). The effect of a national campaign on attitudes toward AIDS. *AIDS Care, 2*(4), 339-346.

Saltzman, L. E., Fanslow, J. L., McMahon, P. M., & Shelley, G. A. (1999). *Intimate partner violence surveillance uniform definitions and recommended data elements.* Atlanta, GA: Center for Disease Control and Prevention.

Sly, D. F, Hopkins, R. S., Trapido, E., & Ray, S. (2001) Influence of a counter advertising media campaign on initiation of smoking: The Florida "truth" campaign. *American Journal of Public Health, 91*(2), 233-38.

Snyder, L. B. (2001). How effective are mediated health campaigns? In R. E. Rice & C. K. Atkin (Eds.), *Public communication campaigns* (pp. 181-192). Thousand Oaks, CA: Sage Publications.

Snyder, L. B., Hamilton, M. A., Mitchell, E. W., Kiwanuka-Yondo, J., Fleming-Milici, F., & Proctor, D. (2004). A meta-analysis of the effect of mediated health communication campaigns on behavior change in the United States. *Journal of Health Communication, 9,* 71-96.

Tjaden, P., & Thoennes, N. (2000). *Extent, nature and consequences of violence against women* (Vol. NCJ-181867). Washington, DC: National Institute of Justice.

U.S. Department of Defense Task Force on Domestic Violence. (2001). *Defense task force on domestic violence year 1 report.* Washington, DC: U.S. Department of Defense.

U.S. Department of Defense Task Force on Domestic Violence. (2002). *Defense task force on domestic violence year 2 report.* Washington, DC: U.S. Department of Defense.

Wallack, L. (1981). Mass media campaigns: The odds against finding behavior change. *Health Education Quarterly, 8*(3), 209-260.

Wallack, L. (1984). Drinking and driving: Toward a broader understanding of a role of the mass media. *Journal of Public Health Policy, 5*(4), 471-496.

Wallack, L., & Dorfman, L. (1996). Media advocacy: A strategy for advancing policy and promoting health. *Health Education Quarterly, 23*(3), 293-317.

Wallack, L., & Dorfman, L. (2001). Putting policy into health communication: The role of media advocacy. In R. E. Rice & C. K. Atkin (Eds.), *Public communication campaigns* (pp. 389-402). Thousand Oaks, CA: Sage Publications.

Weiss, J. A., & Tschirhart, M. (1994). Public information campaigns as policy instruments. *Journal of Policy Analysis and Management, 13*(1), 82-119.

Wilde, G. J. (1993). Effects of mass media communications on health and safety habits: An overview of issues and evidence. *Addiction, 88,* 983-996.

Wilt, S., & Olson, S. (1996). Prevalence of domestic violence in the United States. *Journal of American Women's Medical Association, 51*(3), 77-82.

Wolfe, D. A., & Jaffe, P. G. (1999). Emerging strategies in the prevention of domestic violence. *Future of Children, 9*(3), 133-144.

Wolfe, D. A, Werkele, C., & Scott, K. (1996). *Alternatives to violence: Empowering youth to develop healthy relationships.* Thousand Oaks, CA: Sage.

Woodruff, K. (1996). Alcohol advertising and violence against women: A media advocacy case study. *Health Education Quarterly, 23*(3), 330-345.

Wray, R. J. (2006). Public health communication theory and strategies for interpersonal violence prevention. *Journal of Aggression, Maltreatment & Trauma, 13*(3/4), 41-61.

Wray, R. A., Hornik, R., Gandy, O. H., Stryker, J., Ghez, M., & Mitchell-Clark, K. (2002). *Preventing domestic violence in the African-American community: The impact of a dramatic radio serial.* Unpublished manuscript.

Yanovitzky, I., & Bennett, C. (1999). Media attention, institutional response, and health behavior change: The case of drunk driving, 1987-1999. *Communication Research, 26*(4), 429-453.

Yoder, P. S., Hornik, R., & Chirwa, B. C. (1996). Evaluating the program effects of a radio drama about AIDS in Zambia. *Studies in Family Planning, 27*(4), 188-203.

doi:10.1300/J146v13n03_02

Public Health Communication Theory and Strategies for Interpersonal Violence Prevention

Ricardo J. Wray

SUMMARY. The article reviews experience and lessons learned from public health communication to identify promising strategies for interventions seeking to promote interpersonal violence prevention. A public health perspective highlights multiple levels of analysis in tandem with concomitant communication theory invoking social, institutional, community, and individual change processes. Points of emphasis include a long-term perspective for social change and the importance of achieving high levels of exposure to communication efforts. Alternative communication strategies such as social mobilization, the use of local media, and media advocacy may foster incremental legal reform and service provision, as well as transformed social expectations and norms. doi:10.1300/J146v13n03_03 *[Article copies available for a fee from The Haworth Document Delivery Service: 1-800-HAWORTH. E-mail address: <docdelivery@haworthpress.com> Website: <http://www.HaworthPress.com> © 2006 by The Haworth Press, Inc. All rights reserved.]*

Address correspondence to Dr. Ricardo J. Wray, PhD, Health Communication Research Laboratory, Department of Community Health, School of Public Health, Saint Louis University, 3545 Lafayette Avenue, St. Louis, MO 63104 (E-mail: wray@slu.edu).

[Haworth co-indexing entry note]: "Public Health Communication Theory and Strategies for Interpersonal Violence Prevention." Wray, Ricardo J. Co-published simultaneously in *Journal of Aggression, Maltreatment & Trauma* (The Haworth Maltreatment & Trauma Press, an imprint of The Haworth Press, Inc.) Vol. 13, No. 3/4, 2006, pp. 41-60; and: *Prevention of Intimate Partner Violence* (ed: Sandra M. Stith) The Haworth Maltreatment & Trauma Press, an imprint of The Haworth Press, Inc., 2006, pp. 41-60. Single or multiple copies of this article are available for a fee from The Haworth Document Delivery Service [1-800-HAWORTH, 9:00 a.m. - 5:00 p.m. (EST). E-mail address: docdelivery@haworthpress.com].

KEYWORDS. Interpersonal violence prevention, public health communication, media

Limited evidence from interpersonal violence prevention advocacy groups and public health communication research is suggestive of the potential for communication programs to contribute to prevention initiatives to reduce the incidence of intimate partner violence. A great deal of evidence from the broader research literature in public health communication provides considerable evidence and experience consistent with impact of programs on a variety of behavioral outcomes. This paper draws on the public health and communication literature to identify challenges to and opportunities for developing effective interventions. Specifically, the public health approach to communication invokes multiple levels for analysis and intervention that provide a framework for evaluating theory and evidence. In parallel, the communication literature identifies a set of pathways for communication effects affording opportunities for intervention at multiple levels. The primary aim of this paper is to glean the lessons learned from public health communication research for the ongoing development and assessment of communication interventions that seek to promote domestic violence prevention.

EVIDENCE FROM COMMUNICATION PROGRAMS

Four points stand out in Campbell and Manganello's (this volume) review of mass communication approaches to interpersonal violence prevention as food for thought. First, the authors alert us to the paucity of research about mass media approaches to domestic violence prevention. Second, they note that the few domestic violence prevention interventions that include a mass media component often do not make effective use of behavioral theory. Third, they argue that the experience of communication campaigns in other health behavior areas shows some promise, though campaign impact on average is small. Fourth, they identify a number of important guidelines to bear in mind in developing mass media interventions: consider behavioral complexity; link communication efforts to services, policies and laws; segment audiences and develop media strategies and theory-based messages for these audience segments; and match reasonable program goals with reasonable time frames.

Indeed, the communication literature provides compelling evidence for impact of communication programs, contingent on a variety of factors. Impact has been found for communication programs promoting prevention of HIV, cardiovascular disease, cancer, injuries, and other pressing areas (Hornik, 2002; Institute of Medicine, 2003).

THEORY AND COMMUNICATION PROGRAMS

While behavioral theories are often cited as informing communication campaigns that promote domestic violence prevention, the role of theory has been limited in application (Campbell & Manganello, this volume), or the theories that underlie the campaigns are often not formal or explicit. This is in contrast with research and practice in the broader context of health communication, where theory and evidence are considered essential underpinnings for intervention design and assessment (Hornik, 2002; Maibach & Parrott, 1995; Nelson, Brownson, Remington, & Parvanta, 2003; Rice & Atkin, 1989, 2001). The careful and thoughtful application of theory in communication interventions can be found, to name but a few, in community-based AIDS prevention efforts (e.g., The CDC AIDS Community Demonstration Projects Research Group, 1999), mass media-based smoking cessation programs (Siegel & Biener, 2002; Sly, Heald, & Ray, 2001), and adolescent drug abuse prevention (Cappella, Fishbein, Hornik, Ahern, & Sayeed, 2001).

Why is it important to systematically apply theory in developing communication interventions? As alluded to above, program designers always bring a theoretical understanding of how the world works, but often times these theories take the shape of assumptions about the world, which may mean that programs are designed according to hunches rather than evidence. Social scientific and behavioral theories imply categories of explanation that have been applied and tested in different field and laboratory contexts. Such theories usefully help interventions by enabling us to: explore our assumptions and make them explicit; analyze problems systematically; plan programs and devise reasonable goals; unify program planning and evaluation design; and promote efficiency, effectiveness, and accountability (Glanz, Lewis, & Rimer, 1997).

There is a marked lack of explicit theoretical understanding of behavior in the area of domestic violence prevention, dictating an urgent need for clear definitions and elucidation of target behaviors and their covariates and determinants (Campbell & Manganello, this volume).

The need for a theoretical understanding of domestic violence prevention is of the first order of importance because it bears in every way on how an intervention is designed and evaluated. Our understanding of the target behaviors is directly linked to the nature of the message content of a health promotion effort. Message design is directly connected to our hypotheses, explicit or not, of what underlies a specific behavior. If we think that social norms guide anti-domestic violence behavior, then our campaigns will target social norms. If we think that cognitions such as self-efficacy are most important, then our campaigns will be more individually targeted. If we think law enforcement and service availability count most, then we will attend to these areas first. If we do not think through and test our theories of behavior as an integral part of the intervention planning process, then we are broadcasting aimlessly. Theory-based formative research can help us answer the fundamental question as to whether a communication approach is warranted, or whether other kinds of strategies, such as service provision or policy reform, have greater priority. Among the many theoretical approaches, public health communication offers a useful frame of reference providing perspectives for planning and analysis and opportunities for intervention.

PUBLIC HEALTH APPROACHES TO INTERPERSONAL VIOLENCE PREVENTION

In recent years, the problem of violence has been recast from the legal to the public health domain (Cole & Flanagin, 1998, 1999). By setting violence prevention as a public health priority, national and international health agencies, including the Centers for Disease Control and Prevention (Foege, Rosenberg, & Mercy, 1995), the World Health Organization (World Health Assembly, 1996), and the American Medical Association (Marwick, 1998) have signaled this shift. This reorientation transforms the research we conduct to better understand the problem (Rosenberg, Fenley, Johnson, & Short, 1997; Wallace & Wallace, 1998), and changes the character of the solutions that are proposed to address it (American College of Physicians, 1998; Centers for Disease Control and Prevention, 1997).

Public health practitioners advocate a theoretical approach that distinguishes determinants of behavior, health and illness at social, institutional, community, and individual levels (Stokols, 1992). This overarching viewpoint is consistent with the recommendation that we consider multiple determinants of health in our efforts to safeguard the public's health (Institute of Medicine, 2003). This approach employs a tiered analysis to tease apart the various challenges for best applying public health communication for prevention and reduction of interpersonal violence.

Broadly speaking, theorists distinguish between population and individual level processes or phenomena bearing on health behaviors and outcomes (Jeffery, 1989). For example, the lion's share of health communication programs has historically focused on individual behavior change. The public health perspective highlights the scrutiny we must bring to social and institutional processes, and the potential health benefits we can derive through the judicious application of policy and regulation, and the provision of essential services.

At the same time, communication scholars focus our attention on how we think public communication influences individual, social, and institutional processes and behaviors. Conventional impact assessment generally assumes a direct effect of exposure to communication messages on individual behavior, rather than social or institutional processes. Not surprisingly, linking public communication to access and availability of services in communities, as well as policy and enforcement efforts, enhances the likelihood of impact (Snyder & Hamilton, 2002).

Current communication research recommendations go further than program evaluation to seek to understand how a variety of communication influences affect health behaviors and outcomes (Institute of Medicine, 2003; Smith, 2002). Notably, evaluations of large national behavioral communication interventions have advocated a deeper consideration of indirect effects of communication messages by way of social diffusion and institutional change (Hornik & Yanovitsky, 2003). Whether with regard to intervention design or assessment, the imperative is to integrate multiple individual and social change processes in the theoretical approach that shapes our designs. How can interpersonal violence prevention be construed from the perspective of a multi-level analysis? What are the opportunities at different points of entry for affecting institutions, social networks, and individual behavior in accord with interpersonal violence prevention goals?

ALTERNATIVE EXPLANATIONS OF INTERPERSONAL VIOLENCE PREVENTION

Domestic violence prevention is a set of behaviors only recently taken up by social activists and researchers, so little empirical evidence exists to inform a discussion of potential explanations of behavior. Consequently, while drawing primarily on extant literature, I will also extend approaches to social behavior found in another area, namely, reproductive health. The multi-tiered public health approach contributes useful distinctions between classes of explanations at different levels.

A prominent distinction is often drawn between population (or community or social) and individual level explanations of behavior. In the following discussion, I propose several factors related to interpersonal violence prevention that may be amenable to influence through communication processes at the institutional level, via social or community-level pathways, and finally, via direct effects on individuals.

Social or Community-Level Factors

Institutional or community-level models are based on the assumption that structural factors may constrain or enable individuals to act in desired ways. Thus, even if communication initiatives achieve desired goals of changing specific beliefs and attitudes, behavioral intentions and behavior may not change. It is important to acknowledge community-level factors in individual-level behavior (Jeffery, 1989), such as the presence of legal and social support remedies in the community for domestic violence offenders and victims. To the extent that services are perceived as effective and known to the public, they may incline individuals to seek them out or refer victims to them. In the case of the African American community for example, potential mistrust of law enforcement officials with regard to their behavior toward African American males may limit calls made for assistance (Campbell, Masaki, & Torres, 1997). Entertainment media treatment and press coverage of domestic violence may also influence the extent to which the issue is salient for individuals and lead them to discuss it. On the other hand, media coverage of celebrity athletes convicted of abuse who receive a slap on the wrist and a raise surely contributes to the impression in the general population that domestic violence is not condemned by the community at large.

Other contextual variables may constrain individual behavior, such as the neighborhood in which people live (Mancini et al., this volume). Paquin (1994) argues that neighborhood factors may influence responses to domestic violence. Paquin cites evidence that individuals who know more of their neighbors and are involved in community organizations are more likely to report that they would respond to neighbors' domestic violence. He argues that "Being a parent, married, African American, poor, living in a non-urban area or owning a home predisposes people to have greater contact with their neighbors" (p. 494), and should lead people to respond if they become aware of cases of abuse. This position emphasizes the importance of community context and response. Klein, Campbell, Soler, and Ghez (1997) argue that environmental constraints affect public involvement: "The actions that the public endorses in response to serious violence will be effective only if: Community supports, employment opportunities, and continued protection are provided by the criminal justice system and neighbors to help battered women leave; the total community context enforces batterers' completing long-term treatment; and severe community sanctions are consistently and rigorously imposed against offenders" (p. 62).

Apart from community-level factors, a number of pathways have been posited for how social norms may influence social behavior. One such model underscores the importance of social expectations, which are seen to hinder or support social behaviors. There are two models of effect for this argument. One argues that the proportion of individuals in a community carrying out a behavior will determine the likelihood of other individuals to behave alike, regardless of whether or not they are aware of and can articulate that influence. The second argues that the perception of social expectations is sufficient to affect behavior (Hornik, 1991).

Precipitating community discussion about the topic may stimulate the diffusion of social expectations, or social norms. In setting out to explain determinants of the fertility transition (i.e., adoption of contraception over time, leading to fertility declines), theorists describe specific social behavioral mechanisms that may enhance diffusion. Rosero-Bixby and Casterline (1994) posit three mechanisms: information flow, demonstration effect, and changes in normative context. Bongaarts and Watkins (1997) propose that the exchange of information and ideas, in a context of conversational evaluation, underlies social influence.

Societal expectation models assume that social norms dictate individual behavior, regardless of levels of knowledge or cognitive processes. As the target behaviors for interpersonal violence prevention initiatives are inherently social, existing norms are likely to play a large part in whether or not they are carried out. The social expectation models characterize the fundamental principle that underlies the activities of one leading domestic violence prevention advocacy group, the Family Violence Prevention Fund (FVPF): "In formulating the campaign, our hypothesis was that violence could be reduced by changing the attitudes of the American public about violence against women and by increasing societal involvement in the problem" (Klein et al., 1997, p. xii).

Related to community-level constraints on behavior, individual structural models posit that environmental forces constrain or help behavior. Demographic variables, such as gender, race, culture, and social class, have been found to be influential in whether individuals carry out domestic violence preventive behavior. In a poll carried out for the FVPF, while White and Latino women were found to be significantly more concerned about the growth of domestic violence than men (for Whites, 42% of women, 22% of men; for Latinos, 43% vs. 35% responding "Very worried"), African American men and women expressed the same level of concern, approximately 40% responding "Very worried" (Klein et al., 1997). Greater concern was found among urban and lower income respondents than rural and higher income respondents.

As with the community-level structural models, implicit in the individual structural models is the assumption that structures help or hinder individual behavior. Clearly an interpersonal violence prevention campaign cannot affect the demographics of individuals. However, community characteristics and structures should inform the design and development of culturally targeted interventions.

Individual Level Theories

Communication campaigns frequently build on constructs from a handful of behavioral theories: the Health Belief Model (Rosenstock, 1974), the Theory of Reasoned Action (Ajzen & Fishbein, 1980), Social Cognitive Theory (Bandura, 1986), and the Transtheoretical Model (Prochaska & DiClemente, 1983). A number of texts set out specific techniques for using data from formative audience assessment to effectively tailor messages in a theoretically and empirically sound manner (Cappella et al., 2001; Fishbein, 1995; Hornik & Wolf, 1999; Maibach & Parrott, 1995). Such approaches emphasize program influences on cognitions, such as outcome expectancies and self-efficacy, which are found to influence behavior in audience surveys. Behavioral theorists agree on the importance of being very specific about risk behaviors, defining them operationally in terms of situation, context, and time, and so facilitating programmatic application and measurement (Fishbein, 1995). Formative and summative research has identified cognitive factors associated with interpersonal violence prevention behaviors, including issue salience, outcome expectations, and self-efficacy (Wray, Hornik, Gandy, Stryker, Ghez, & Mitchell-Clark, 2004).

Behaviorist models assume that, all things being equal, individuals will only carry out behaviors if they expect to be rewarded (Hornik, 1991). The nature of the behaviors of interest would suggest possible constraints prompted by this model. There may be a potential perceived threat of real danger, in the case of speaking with an abused woman (Klein et al., 1997). Depicting appropriate conversational tactics, providing information about where help can be sought and emphasizing the potential benefits for victims can counter fear of repercussions. Speaking out about domestic violence may be indicative of community concern and garner the speaker respect, or it may result in accusations of naïveté by the more cynical. If an intervention promotes social norms supportive of the notion of the unacceptability of domestic violence, the latter threat may be diminished.

Affect and emotional reactions are important precursors to motivation, which can lead to behavior (Hornik, 1991). The issue of domestic violence may lead some listeners to fear taking steps if they learn of or witness an incident. Interpersonal violence prevention efforts may provide important information regarding what kind of safe steps may be taken to counter this fear. They may help to reinforce the salience of the issue, already found to be at high levels among Americans (Klein et al., 1997).

Conclusion

A variety of factors have been found to be associated with the likelihood that people will take steps to prevent interpersonal violence, such as speaking to a victim of domestic violence, or in general about the subject. Conversations are manifestly social behaviors, and as such are especially threatened by traditional social norms that domestic violence is a private matter. However, diffusion of social norms can run both ways. In the case of the diffusion of fertility related norms, ideas that ran counter to family planning early on in the fertility transition were transformed and later supported family planning (Bongaarts & Watkins, 1997). The long run goal of interpersonal violence prevention strategies should be to transform social norms with relation to community response to domestic violence. Klein et al. (1997) cite the gradual but unequivocal changes in attitudes about smoking and drunk driving over time as the model of social change they seek to elicit.

It is clear that institutional, community-level, social, and individual factors may restrict or enhance the effectiveness of the interpersonal violence prevention efforts. Perceptions about institutions, such as medical services and law enforcement, can influence the likelihood of individuals to seek assistance. Neighborhood embeddedness and family structure seem to be a strong determinant of social support, and social interaction may well shape social norms. Cognitive factors appear to account for individual behavior to some degree.

This review is based on the premise that public communication programs need to take into account challenges and opportunities at all levels. By establishing an empirical basis for multiple determinants of interpersonal violence prevention behaviors, a multi-faceted communication strategy can be strategically brought to bear. The next section offers examples of approaches for intervention that aim to galvanize social diffusion and institutional change strategies, as well as raise awareness and shape expectancy and efficacy beliefs at the individual level.

PUBLIC COMMUNICATION APPROACHES

Primary goals of the domestic violence prevention community have been to offer shelter and services to victims, as well as to influence how courts, enforcement agencies, and other policy actors respond to incidents of abuse (Rosenberg et al., 1997). An emerging perspective adopts an analytical approach informed by public health models that emphasize the social and cultural contexts of abuse, and highlight prevention in addition to treatment (Cole & Flanagin, 1998). Among other approaches, such as mandatory alternative treatment for batterers and professional training for service providers who come into contact with victims, this perspective is increasingly reflected in communication interventions that are designed to change beliefs, norms, and social practices related to abuse (Rosenberg et al., 1997). The public health model also highlights the role of evaluation in testing the effectiveness of new and alternative interventions (Rosenberg et al., 1997).

Proponents of domestic violence prevention activities suggest that above and beyond the important efforts to influence the behavior of abusers and victims, successful interventions must also address the social norms, beliefs, and practices related to domestic violence among the individuals living around and interacting with those directly involved in abuse. Both advocates and researchers argue that transforming social norms from those of silence and toleration to intervention and condemnation is essential to the long-term reduction of domestic violence (Klein et al., 1997; Rosenberg et al., 1997). Much as shelters provide a safe space for battered women to regroup and regain their self-confidence, activation of a social support network can "simulate the shelter experience through group work embodying the principles of recovery, safety, support, and empowerment . . . The social support a woman musters often holds the key to whether she can be both safe and separate" (Stark & Flitcraft, 1996, pp. 178-179). How can public communication contribute to this effort?

THE IMPORTANCE OF EXPOSURE

Recent studies have demonstrated that reach of a campaign is directly linked to its potential for success at the population level (Snyder & Hamilton, 2002). Such findings have led to a call for a shift in research focus from an emphasis in the health communication literature on behavioral theory and message design (Maibach & Parrott, 1995) towards a better understanding of exposure (Hornik, 2002). This is not to say that the importance of behavioral theory should be under-estimated, but to give equivalent emphasis to theories of campaign effects and strategies of message dissemination.

The most impeccably designed interventions, no matter how soundly based in theory, will go nowhere without achieving sufficient reach in the desired audience. Achieving adequate reach must be a central strategic goal in any intervention, including mass media campaigns. While this point may seem self-evident, it is surprisingly often overlooked. Inadequate exposure has been identified as a weakness in community-control studies, in which the avoidance of contamination in the control communities and the demands of study design overshadow requirements of exposure (Hornik, 2002). Exposure can also be an issue in the context of public service campaigns that depend on the good will of broadcasters to donate airtime (DeJong & Winsten, 1998; Institute of Medicine, 2003). Put bluntly, exposure is a function of expenditure–of time and money.

To make this point clear, two cautionary tales of interpersonal violence prevention campaigns are presented (Stryker, Hornik, Wray, & Appleyard, 2000; Wray et al., 2004). Both interventions were implemented by the FVPF and evaluated by a team at the Annenberg School for Communication at the University of Pennsylvania, led by Dr. Robert

Hornik. The theoretical approach for both campaigns was based on the model introduced by the Fund: preventing domestic violence by changing social norms from tolerance to condemnation. In addition, the campaigns provided information about specific actions that individuals could take to intervene on behalf of victims.

The "Philadelphia: Let's Stop Domestic Violence" Campaign set out to raise awareness and prompt community action about the issue through social mobilization in neighborhoods and through media advocacy. The "It's Your Business" Campaign sought to reach African American adults through a radio serial drama that told a story about a community helping a woman who was being abused by her husband. Both campaigns were theory driven and carefully evaluated. And both campaigns ended up hampered by limited exposure. Evidence for limited short-term effects was found in the Philadelphia case. In the case of the "It's Your Business" campaign, we found evidence of an association between campaign exposure and anti-domestic violence beliefs, attitudes, and behaviors. However, exposure levels were so low that we concluded that this association was more likely due to selective exposure than to campaign impact (i.e., the causal order was reversed). The "It's Your Business" campaign in particular was a good example of a theoretically and empirically informed message design. Unfortunately, we were not able to fairly evaluate the campaigns, as so few people in the audiences were exposed to them.

The lessons we learned from these two experiences focused on the challenge of achieving exposure in the public service context for domestic violence prevention activities. The innovative efforts made by the FVPF aimed to attract the attention of the press (in the case of the Philadelphia campaign) and African American radio stations (in the context of the radio serial), and both failed. We learned that media advocacy requires a particular set of circumstances to increase the likelihood of success. The radio serial may not have worked because of the length of each segment, or because of the topic. The question remains, how can we garner attention for the issue, in the public service context, short of paying for it?

ALTERNATIVE COMMUNICATION STRATEGIES

Communication interventions have become increasingly sophisticated, incorporating approaches aiming to influence policy, provoke discussion, and affect behavior with a variety of strategies in the toolkit of programmers. Above and beyond an understanding of behavioral determinants, communication experts need to think through the possible avenues of influence of public communication programs. This more nuanced understanding of communication processes incorporates the potential for direct individual level effects, as well as indirect effects via social diffusion and institutional change (Hornik & Yanovitzky, 2003).

Contemporary thinking regarding communication interventions extends beyond the domain of mass media campaigns targeting individual behavior, to community level programs requiring a thoughtful consideration of social and institutional processes. In addition to the targeted use of media, public health practitioners may wield a range of interventions that seek to account for the multiple determinants of health behaviors and outcomes. Consistent with classical approaches to communication, interventions should be informed by behavioral theory, as well as representing well thought out expectations and theories of program effects. At the same time, communication initiatives should be linked vertically, connecting appropriately to services and raising awareness about law enforcement programs. The interpersonal violence prevention community needs to think strategically and plan for the long-term, and bear in mind the painstaking work that has contributed to the decline of drunk driving and smoking over decades. Several alternative strategies hold promise. The balance of the paper introduces a few examples.

Social Mobilization

While broadly conceived as a public health strategy, social mobilization includes critical elements consistent with public communication approaches. Such strategies acknowledge the crucial role of the neighborhood and social network in guiding or obstructing social behaviors. Social mobilization approaches include recruitment, training, and empowerment of community leaders, as has been effectively applied in the context of family planning programs in Bangladesh (Kincaid, 2000) and HIV prevention work in this country (Fisher, 1988). Social mobilization strategies also tap into advances in social theory, emphasizing the importance of community-level factors. Researchers have capitalized on the notion of collective efficacy (Bandura, 1997) in implementing community development initiatives aiming to promote pro-social behavior among inner city youth (Sampson, Raudenbush, & Earls, 1997). Allocation of funding for programs may go in this vein to support local initiatives to foster organizational growth and development.

A novel project using this approach in the area of violence prevention has recently achieved considerable success. The Ceasefire project in Chicago has implemented a community-level strategy to shift social norms around the use of handguns. The approach has emphasized organizational strategies, providing training and resources to individuals and institutions at the neighborhood level to affect the context in which violence takes place. In addition to the organizational work, the project has also made use of limited mass media approaches, in the form of publicity visible at the neighborhood level. The project has successfully reduced the level of mortality due to handguns in target neighborhoods, compared to controls (Robert Wood Johnson Foundation, 2003).

The limitation of such an approach lies in its necessarily small scope. The challenge is to establish guidelines to support existing neighborhood advocacy and development groups to adopt pro-social programs. An empirical question remains–how can neighborhood organizations take advantage of, or link into, national or regional mass media campaigns promoting parallel goals?

Local or Mini-Media

An alternative approach to the more diffuse and necessarily generalized approach of a large-scale media campaign is the idea of supporting small-scale and local communication initiatives. Such efforts have been credited with success in HIV and violence prevention efforts (Green, Nantulya, Stoneburner, & Stover, 2002; Robert Wood Johnson Foundation, 2003; Slutkin, 2000).

The unparalleled success of HIV prevention efforts in Uganda has prompted a great deal of analysis of the factors that contributed to the decline of HIV prevalence there; no other country on the continent has experienced any comparable decline. One factor that has been seen to contribute to the success has been the allocation of communication and prevention resources at the local or municipal level. This decentralized approach to planning and implementation for communication programs was able to reach general audiences as well as key target groups. This management model has allowed the creation of locally generated communication materials. Such materials, created by and for people within the target area, can be both visible and pertinent for the population, and may prove to contribute to behavior change despite adverse circumstances such as conflict and poverty (Green et al., 2002; Slutkin, 2000).

This approach has two unique requirements: devolved funding to the local level and heightened local relevance. At the same time, the approach poses challenges to the public health advocate, given that local autonomy in message design can sometimes achieve results that run counter to national campaign messages or goals. However, local relevance and effectiveness should trump national rhetorical strategies. More work needs to be done to assess how local community initiatives can best tap into and leverage national media initiatives.

Media Advocacy and News

Apart from the need for continued efforts on the part of public health practitioners and interpersonal violence prevention advocates to design, implement, and assess deliberate communication interventions, it is also crucial to continue to sensitize the news media on the issue. Practitioners and advocates cultivate ongoing relationships with writers and editors from the news media in order to make sure that the interpersonal violence prevention agenda gets a fair hearing from the news media.

Public health researchers have included the idea of media advocacy as an important strategy to harness the media in efforts to affect public policy (Wallack & Dorfman, 1996). This approach acknowledges that the way stories are framed affects both whether news sources will pick them up for inclusion, and the extent to which they may influence public and political perceptions (Wallack, Woodruff, Dorfman, & Diaz, 1999). Agenda setting theory posits that news media can influence public opinion as well as policy agendas (McCombs & Reynolds, 2002). A promising strategy for influencing the agenda of local news media is to highlight the local angle of a national story (Wallack et al., 1999). This approach is also consistent with political communication theory, which implicates the local media as vital participants in the articulation of issues like interpersonal violence prevention. An active media contributes to ongoing debate about issues, and may potentially lead to heightened participation by citizens in advocacy for policy change (Friedland & McLeod, 1999).

All these strategies may be seen as having the potential to contribute to a gradual shift of norms and beliefs over time. By applying multiple tactical approaches and strategic objectives, interpersonal violence prevention advocates can plan fundamental change of institutional practices, social norms, and individual beliefs and behaviors in the long-term. In any single time period, however, only incremental shifts should be expected.

Evaluation: What About the Secular Trend?

The experience of research and practice with communication interventions shows promise for the prevention of domestic violence, assuming we design programs based on an explicit theoretical understanding of behavior and campaign effects. Three areas of continued research appear especially pressing. First, it is incumbent on us to develop and test theory-based mechanisms for domestic violence prevention. Second, we must continue to explore avenues for gaining maximal exposure and accounting for multiple levels of influence. Third, we must be aware of trade-offs between exposure and rigor in evaluation design.

Public health interventions do not happen in a vacuum. Substantial national trends in health behaviors sometimes overtake public health campaigns and research about them. Many of the most expensive studies of strategies seeking to influence health behaviors, using the best theory and design that science has to offer, have resulted in little or no impact, due to the substantial change found in the control communities. Two prominent examples of this are the Stanford Five Community Study (Farquhar et al., 1990), and the Community Intervention Trial for Smoking Cessation trial (COMMIT; 1995). One explanation for these results is that there was very little real exposure to the campaigns in the target populations, or very little difference in exposure levels between the intervention and control communities. This experience stands in contrast to large national campaigns that appear to have shown remarkable influence on health behavior, such as the National High Blood Pressure Education Program (NHBPEP; Roccella, 2002). A meta-analysis of 48 communication campaigns found a strong link ($r = .47$) between level of exposure to a campaign and likelihood of impact (Snyder & Hamilton, 2002).

The issue arises that in multifaceted campaigns of the scale of the NHBPEP, it is impossible to unequivocally attribute behavior change to them. There is an inherent tension between the potential for impact and the requirements of study design in the capacity for a campaign to achieve substantial exposure. Though they lack the conditional rigor of randomized controlled trials, some quasi-experimental study designs can provide sufficient and suggestive evidence of impact, and not thwart efforts to gain maximal exposure. Studies can effectively reduce uncertainty about program impact if they incorporate measurement at multiple time points, compare exposed and unexposed populations, establish that effects are consistent with theoretical models, triangulate evidence, and focus on audience segments (Hornik, 2002).

ARE SMALL EFFECTS ENOUGH?

It is important to remember that at the population level, a few percentage points translate into large numbers of people (Sorensen, Emmons, Hunt, & Johnston, 1998). Epidemiologist Geoffrey Rose (1992) introduced the notion of the Prevention Paradox, when he argued that shifting the population a little bit on important behaviors has a greater impact on health outcomes than shifting only those individuals most at risk a great deal. This is true in the case of chronic disease like cancer and heart disease, and in the link between nutritional status and susceptibility to mortality due to infection. It may be that the same argument can also be made for domestic violence prevention. Incremental changes in institutions in the shape of legal reform and service provision, as well as transformed social expectations and norms may prove to have a greater effect in reducing interpersonal violence in the long haul than strategies that target victims and perpetrators. Such primary prevention approaches should at the very least be seen as requisite adjuncts to programs that seek to influence intimate partners themselves.

REFERENCES

Ajzen, I., & Fishbein, M. (1980). *Understanding attitudes and predicting social behavior*. Englewood Cliffs, NJ: Prentice Hall.

American College of Physicians. (1998). Firearm injury prevention: Clinical guidelines. *Annals of Internal Medicine, 128*(3), 236-41.

Bandura, A. (1986). *Social foundations of thought and action*. Englewood Cliffs, NJ: Prentice Hall.

Bandura, A. (1997). *Self-efficacy*. New York: WH Freeman and Co.

Bongaarts, J., & Watkins, S. C. (1996). Social interactions and contemporary fertility transitions. *Population and Development Review, 22*(4), 639-682, 813, 815-816.

Campbell, D. W., Masaki, B., & Torres, S. (1997). Water on rock: Changing domestic violence perceptions in the African American, Asian American and Latino communities. In E. Klein, J. Campbell, E. Soler, & M. Ghez (Eds.), *Ending domestic violence* (pp. 64-87). Thousand Oaks, CA: Sage.

Campbell, J. C., & Manganello, J. (2006). Changing public attitudes as a prevention strategy to reduce intimate partner violence. *Journal of Aggression, Maltreatment & Trauma, 12*(2/3), 13-19.

Cappella, J. N., Fishbein, M., Hornik, R., Ahern, R. K., & Sayeed, S. (2001). Using theory to select messages in anti-drug media campaigns. In R. E. Rice & C. K. Atkin (Eds.), *Public communication campaigns* (3rd ed., pp. 214-230). Thousand Oaks, CA: Sage.

CDC AIDS Community Demonstration Projects Research Group. (1999). Community-level HIV intervention in five cities: Final outcome data from the CDC AIDS

Community Demonstration Projects. *American Journal of Public Health,* 89(3), 336-345.

Centers for Disease Control and Prevention. (1997). Perceptions of child sexual abuse as a public health problem–Vermont September 1995. *Morbidity and Mortality Weekly Report, 46*(34), 801-803.

Cole, T. B., & Flanagin, A. (1998). Violence–ubiquitous, threatening and preventable. *The Journal of the American Medical Association, 280*(5), 468.

Cole, T. B., & Flanagin, A. (1999). What can we do about violence? *The Journal of the American Medical Association, 282*(5), 481.

Community Intervention Trial for Smoking Cessation. (1995). I. Cohort results from a four year intervention. *American Journal of Public Health, 85,* 183-192.

Dejong, W., & Winsten, J. (1998). *The media and the message: Lessons learned from past public service campaigns.* Washington, DC: The National Campaign to Prevent Teen Pregnancy.

Farquhar, J. W., Fortmann, S. P., Flora, J. A., Taylor, C. B., Haskell, W. L., Williams, P. T. et al. (1990). Effects of communitywide education on cardiovascular disease risk factors. The Stanford Five City Project. *Journal of the American Medical Association, 264*(3), 359-365.

Fishbein, M. (1995). Developing effective behavior change interventions: Some lessons learned from behavioral research. In T. E. Backer, S. L. David, & G. Soucy (Eds.), *Reviewing the behavioral science knowledge base on technology transfer* (NIDA Monographs No. 155, pp. 246-261). Rockville, MD: National Institute on Drug Abuse.

Fisher, J. D. (1988). Possible effects of reference group-based social influence on AIDS-risk behavior and AIDS prevention. *American Psychologist, 43*(11), 914-920.

Foege, W. H., Rosenberg, M. L., & Mercy, J. A. (1995). Public health and violence prevention. *Current Issues in Public Health, 1,* 2-9.

Friedland, L. A., & McLeod, J. M. (1999). Community integration and mass media: A reconsideration. In D. Demers & K. Viswanath (Eds.), *Mass media, social control, and social change: A macro-social perspective* (pp. 197-228). Ames, IA: Iowa State University Press.

Glanz, K., Lewis, F., & Rimer, B. (1997). *Health behavior and health education* (2nd ed.). San Francisco: Jossey Bass.

Green, E., Nantulya, V., Stoneburner, R., & Stover, J. (2002). *What happened in Uganda? Declining HIV prevalence, behavior change, and the national response.* Washington, DC: USAID.

Hornik, R. (1991). Alternative models of behavior change. In J. Wasserheit, S. Aral, K. Holmes, & P. Hitchcock (Eds.), *Research issues in human behavior and sexually transmitted diseases in the AIDS era* (pp. 210-217). Washington, DC: American Society for Microbiology.

Hornik, R. (Ed). (2002). *Public health communication: evidence for behavior change.* Mahwah, NJ: Lawrence Erlbaum.

Hornik, R., & Wolf, K. (1999). Using cross-sectional surveys to plan message strategies. *Social Marketing Quarterly, 5,* 34-41.

Hornik, R., & Yanovitzky, I. (2003). Using theory to design evaluations of communication campaigns: The case of the National Youth Anti-Drug Media Campaign. *Communication Theory, 13*(2), 204-224.

Institute of Medicine. (2003). *The future of the public's health in the 21st century.* Washington DC: The National Academies Press.

Jeffery, R. (1989). Risk behaviors and health: Contrasting individual and population perspectives. *American Psychologist, 44*(9), 1194-1202.

Kincaid, D. L. (2000). Social networks, ideation, and contraceptive behavior in Bangladesh: A longitudinal analysis. *Social Science & Medicine, 50*(2), 215-31.

Klein, E., Campbell, J., Soler, E., & Ghez, M. (1997). *Ending domestic violence.* Thousand Oaks, CA: Sage.

Maibach, E., & Parrot, R. L. (Eds.) (1995). *Designing health messages: Approaches from communication theory and public health practice.* Thousand Oaks, CA: Sage.

Mancini, J. A., Nelson, J. P., Bowen, G., & Martin, J. A. (2006). Preventing intimate partner violence: A community capacity approach. *Journal of Aggression, Maltreatment & Trauma, 12*(2/3), 203-227.

Marwick, C. (1998). Domestic violence recognized as a world problem. *The Journal of the American Medical Association, 279*(19), 1510.

McCombs, M., & Reynolds, A. (2002). News influence on our pictures of the world. In J. Bryant & D. Zillman (Eds.), *Media effects: Advances in theory and research* (pp. 1-18). Mahwah, NJ: Erlbaum and Associates.

Nelson, D. E., Brownson, R. C., Remington, P. L., & Parvanta, C. (2002). *Communicating public health information effectively.* Washington, DC: APHA.

Paquin, G. W. (1994). A statewide survey of reactions to neighbors' domestic violence. *Journal of Interpersonal Violence, 9*(4), 493-502.

Prochaska, J. O., & DiClemente, C. C. (1983). Stages and processes of self-change of smoking: Toward an integrative model of change. *Journal of Consulting and Clinical Psychology, 51*(3), 390-395.

Rice, R., & Atkin, C. (1989). *Public communication campaigns* (2nd ed.). Newbury Park, CA: Sage.

Rice, R., & Atkin, C. (2001). *Public communication campaigns* (3rd ed.). Thousand Oaks, CA: Sage.

Robert Wood Johnson Foundation. (2003). *Treating violence as a contagious disease.* Retrieved July 9, 2003 from http://www.rwjf.org/news/profiles/slutkin_1.jhtml

Roccella, E. J. (2002). The contributions of public health education toward the reduction of cardiovascular disease mortality: Experiences from the National High Blood Pressure Education Program. In R. Hornik (Ed.), *Public health communication: Evidence for behavior change* (pp. 73-84). Mahwah, NJ: Lawrence Erlbaum.

Rose, G. (1992). *Strategy of preventive medicine.* Oxford: Oxford University Press.

Rosenberg, M. L., Fenley, M. A., Johnson, D., & Short, L. (1997). Bridging prevention and practice: Public health and family violence. *Academic Medicine, 72*(1, Suppl.), S13-18.

Rosenstock, I. M. (1974). Historical origins of the health belief model. In M. H. Becker (Ed.), *The health belief model and personal health behavior* (pp. 1-8). Thorofare, NH: Charles B. Slack.

Rosero-Bixby, L., & Casterline, J.B. (1994). Interaction diffusion and fertility transition in Costa Rica. *Social Forces, 73*(2), 435-462.

Sampson, R. J., Raudenbush, S. W., & Earls, F. (1997). Neighborhoods and violent crime: A multi-level study of collective efficacy. *Science, 277*(5328), 918-924.

Siegel, M., & Biener, L. (2002). The impact of anti-smoking media campaigns on progression to established smoking: Results of a longitudinal youth study in Massachusetts. In R. Hornik (Ed.), *Public health communication: Evidence for behavior change* (pp. 115-130). Mahwah, NJ: Lawrence Erlbaum.

Slutkin, G. (2000). Global AIDS 1981-1999: The response. *International Journal of Tuberculosis & Lung Disease, 4*(2 Suppl 1), S24-33.

Sly, D. F., Heald, G. R., & Ray, S. (2001). The Florida "truth" anti-tobacco media evaluation: Design, first year results, and implications for planning future state media evaluations. *Tobacco Control, 10*, 9-15.

Smith, W. (2002). From prevention *vaccines* to community care: New ways to look at program success. In R. Hornik (Ed.), *Public health communication: Evidence for behavior change* (pp. 327-356). Mahwah, NJ: Lawrence Erlbaum.

Snyder, L., & Hamilton, M. (2002). A meta-analysis of US health campaign effects on behavior: Emphasize enforcement, exposure, and new information, and beware the secular trend. In R. Hornik (Ed.), *Public health communication: Evidence for behavior change* (pp. 357-383). Mahwah, NJ: Lawrence Erlbaum.

Sorensen, G., Emmons, K., Hunt, M. K., & Johnston, D. (1998). Implications of the results of community intervention trials. *Annual Review of Public Health, 19*, 379-416.

Stark, E., & Flitcraft, A. (1996). *Women at risk: Domestic violence and women's health.* Thousand Oaks, CA: Sage Publications.

Stokols, D. (1992). Establishing and maintaining healthy environments: Toward a social ecology of health promotion. *American Psychologist, 47*(1), 6-22.

Stryker, J., Hornik, R., Wray, R., & Appleyard, J. (2000). *Media advocacy and social mobilization to reduce domestic violence: The evaluation of the Philadelphia: Let's Stop Domestic Violence! Campaign.* Presented at the Annual Meeting of the International Communication Association, Acapulco, Mexico.

Wallace, D., & Wallace, R. (1998). Scales of geography, time and population: The study of violence as a public health problem. *American Journal of Public Health, 88*(12), 1853-1858.

Wallack, L., & Dorfman, L. (1996). Media advocacy: A strategy for advancing policy and promoting health. *Health Education Quarterly, 23*(3), 293-317.

Wallack, L., Woodruff, K., Dorfman, L., & Diaz, I. (1999). *News for a change: An advocate's guide to working with the media.* Thousand Oaks, CA: Sage.

World Health Assembly. (1996). WHA 49.25 Resolution: Prevention of violence: A public health priority. *49th World Health Assembly, Geneva, Switzerland,* 20-25 May.

Wray, R., Hornik, R., Gandy, O., Stryker, J., Ghez, M., & Mitchell-Clark, K. (2004). Preventing domestic violence in the African American community: Assessing the impact of a dramatic radio serial. *Journal of Health Communication, 9*(1), 31-52.

doi:10.1300/J146v13n03_03

CHANGING THE WAY
THE HEALTH CARE SYSTEM RESPONDS
TO INTIMATE PARTNER VIOLENCE

Domestic Violence Screening
in Medical and Mental Health Care Settings:
Overcoming Barriers
to Screening, Identifying, and Helping
Partner Violence Victims

L. Kevin Hamberger
Mary Beth Phelan

SUMMARY. Health care providers and patients agree that domestic violence presents a serious health issue that falls within the purview of medical care. The patient-physician encounter has the potential to assist domestic violence victims in considering their options of living without

Address correspondence to L. Kevin Hamberger, PhD, Racine Family Practice Center, P.O. Box 548, Racine, WI 53401-0548 (E-Mail: lkh@mcw.edu).

[Haworth co-indexing entry note]: "Domestic Violence Screening in Medical and Mental Health Care Settings: Overcoming Barriers to Screening, Identifying, and Helping Partner Violence Victims." Hamberger, L. Kevin, and Mary Beth Phelan. Co-published simultaneously in *Journal of Aggression, Maltreatment & Trauma* (The Haworth Maltreatment & Trauma Press, an imprint of The Haworth Press, Inc.) Vol. 13, No. 3/4, 2006, pp. 61-99; and: *Prevention of Intimate Partner Violence* (ed: Sandra M. Stith) The Haworth Maltreatment & Trauma Press, an imprint of The Haworth Press, Inc., 2006, pp. 61-99. Single or multiple copies of this article are available for a fee from The Haworth Document Delivery Service [1-800-HAWORTH, 9:00 a.m. - 5:00 p.m. (EST). E-mail address: docdelivery@haworthpress.com].

violence and playing a critical role in preventing future violence. Despite this possibility, many persons evaluated in the health care system do not experience the benefits of such interactions. This article reviews current research that evaluates physician, patient, and systems barriers to providing care to patients experiencing domestic violence as well as gaps in the current research and suggestions for how these barriers might be overcome. Educational initiatives, implementation of protocols, and increasing environmental cues that prompt patients and physicians to discuss domestic violence may all increase the likelihood of screening and the success of interventions. doi:10.1300/J146v13n03_04 *[Article copies available for a fee from The Haworth Document Delivery Service: 1-800-HAWORTH. E-mail address: <docdelivery@haworthpress.com> Website: <http://www.HaworthPress.com> © 2006 by The Haworth Press, Inc. All rights reserved.]*

KEYWORDS. Domestic violence, health care screening, barriers to domestic violence screening

Over the past several years, there has been an explosion of research into the issue of family violence as a public health problem for which health care professionals and providers have a legitimate role for intervention and prevention (Burge, 1989; Koop & Lundberg, 1992). This has not always been the case. Hendricks-Matthews (1991), for example, found that only 36% of family practice residency programs responding to a survey provided any type of training on domestic violence. Further, only 14% of family practice residency program directors even believed that residency programs should be greatly involved in teaching about violence. Sugg and Inui (1992) reported that 61% of practicing physicians in their study did not receive violence education, either during medical school, residency, or during continuing education as a professional. Health professionals have consistently reported lack of education as a major barrier to screening, identifying, and helping partner violence victims in health care settings.

Since the mid-1980s, Surgeons General have spearheaded national efforts to raise physician awareness of violence, particularly domestic violence, as a public health problem requiring a multidisciplinary approach (Novello, 1992; Surgeon General, 1985). In addition to the efforts of the surgeons general, major medical associations have published policy statements and guidelines for identifying and helping victims of partner violence. These include the American Medical Association (AMA; 1992), American College of Emergency Physicians (1995), American Academy of Pediatrics, (1998), and the American College of Obstetrics and Gynecology (1989, 2000).

Research clearly shows that, throughout the health care system, prevalence of women struggling with the impact of domestic violence, both in their current relationships and during their lifetime, is high (Abbott, Johnson, Koziol-McLain, & Lowenstein, 1995; Hamberger, Saunders, & Hovey, 1992; McGrath, Hogan, & Piepert, 1998). Further, the research suggests that domestic violence exacts a tremendous impact on victims and survivors, both in terms of physical and mental health problems, and health care costs (Cascardi, Langhinrichsen, & Vivian, 1992; Coben, Forjuoh, & Gondolf, 1999). Moreover, compared to nonbattered women, battered women appear to exhibit a number of fairly consistent risk markers. Some of these risk markers are related to physical and mental health profiles (Crowell & Burgess, 1996; Saunders, Hamberger, & Hovey, 1993). Others are related to demographics, such as age and marital status (Hamberger et al., 1992; Wilt & Olson, 1996). It would stand to reason, therefore, that developing systematic, effective means for screening and identifying such patients appears to be potentially beneficial for both providers and patients. Once identified, providers would offer abuse victims and survivors adequate support and information to facilitate their healing process, prevent future violence, and ultimately end the violence in their lives. In fact, health care providers frequently feel sympathy for battered victims, acknowledge the importance of domestic violence as a health care issue, and agree that health care providers both have much to offer and must be involved in identifying and helping domestic violence victims as part of their practice (Coleman & Stith, 1997; Eastel & Eastel, 1992). Both patients and physicians generally view domestic violence as a legitimate health problem (Friedman, Samet, Roberts, Hudlin, & Hans, 1992). However, research suggests that, while many patients and physicians are willing to discuss domestic violence, many more are not (Friedman et al., 1992; Hayden, Barton, & Hayden, 1997).

Other data suggest that health care providers frequently do a poor job of screening for domestic violence; reported screening rates among family physicians range from 1.7% to 4% (Hamberger et al., 1992; Rath, Jarratt, & Leonardson, 1989), and similar low rates of screening have been found in emergency departments (Stark, Flitcraft, & Frazier, 1979) and maternal health care settings (Hillard, 1985). More recently, Rodriguez, Bauer, McLoughlin, and Grumbach (1999) reported that, among primary care physicians, only 10% reported routine screening with new patients, 9% screened during routine, periodic checkups, and

11% routinely screened during prenatal visits. Clark et al. (2000) showed that 37% of the respondents reported having been screened during prenatal care.

Despite the need and the potential for healthcare providers to play an active role in prevention and intervention into domestic violence, there is little evidence that they are doing so in large numbers or in systematic ways. Yet healthcare providers are in a position to assist victims in considering their options of living without violence, and to play a critical role in preventing future violence. This article reviews the literature on barriers to helping victims in health care settings, as well has how to best address and overcome them. The primary aim of the article is to provide a critical review of the literature in this area, describing the state of the research as well as gaps in our current knowledge base and methodological problems posed by current research. Critical reviews can leave the impression that insufficient evidence exists to warrant clinical application. However, given the acute need in health care to provide important, often life saving services to partner violence victims, implications of the research for clinical practice will also be discussed.

BARRIERS TO SCREENING AND IDENTIFICATION

Health care providers and patients face many barriers to screening, identifying, and helping patients who are involved in violent intimate relationships. In general, these barriers can be identified at various levels of the health care intervention process. These include barriers unique to the health care provider, barriers that lie with the patient, and barriers that are created or maintained by the overall health care system. In addition, some barriers seem to emerge from the nature of the interaction between provider and patient.

Healthcare Provider Barriers

Within the provider-patient relationship, health care providers play an important role in facilitating or impeding appropriate assessment, diagnosis, and treatment. An important component of the assessment and diagnostic process involves clinical interviewing techniques and strategies, as well as clinical observation. A number of factors can impede clinician efforts to gather information.

Lack of Knowledge. Perhaps the most typically identified barrier is lack of education (Sugg & Inui, 1992). Among their sample of 38 primary care physicians, 61% reported not having had previous training in domestic violence. Thirty-two percent of Canadian primary care physicians (Ferris, 1994) and 71% of obstetrician-gynecologists (Parsons, Zaccaro, Wells, & Stovall, 1995) as well as 68% of dentists (Love, Gerbert, Caspers, Bronstone, Perry, & Bird, 2001) cited lack of training as a major barrier to screening. Hamberger, Guse, Boerger, Minske, Pape, and Folsom (2004) found that nearly 50% of nursing staff (n = 752), with an average career duration of 14 years, working at a community-based medical system did not have prior training in domestic violence. Although, in recent years, more medical schools and residency programs have developed and included family violence curricula (Hendricks-Matthews, 1991), such training is variable in terms of quantity and quality. Significant training gaps persist, leaving health care providers unprepared to screen, identify, and help partner violence victims.

No research has been published on the precise training and knowledge gaps that prevent clinicians from screening for domestic violence. For some providers, domestic violence is "not on the radar screen," so they may assume that their communities and patients do not have such problems (Parsons et al., 1995; Moore, Zaccaro, & Parsons, 1998). Some providers may possess knowledge about domestic violence, but lack skill in how to ask about it and facilitate valid responses. No studies were found that evaluated the actual skill with which providers ask about domestic violence. A third area of knowledge and skill deficit is in performing the complex set of responses to patients who either acknowledge living in an abusive relationship or show many positive signs of doing so, but deny it. Providers frequently object to screening on the basis that they will not know what to say or do if a patient responds to screening in the affirmative (Ferris, 1994). Another knowledge-base area that frequently vexes health care providers is whether they have a duty to report partner abuse to authorities. Several states have laws that specifically mandate health care reporters to report domestic violence to authorities, and some states also require reporting of children exposed to intimate partner violence. Almost all other states have laws that require health care professionals to report injuries related to crime (Hyman, Schillinger, & Lo, 1995). However, health care providers are frequently reluctant to make such reports due to concerns about patient autonomy, as well as damage to the provider-patient relationship (Rodriguez et al., 1999).

Fear of Offending Patients. Another frequently mentioned barrier to screening and helping abuse victims experienced by health care providers is fear that their patients will be offended when asked about domestic abuse (Moore et al., 1998; Sugg & Inui, 1992). National surveys of obstetrician-gynecologists (Parsons et al., 1995) and dentists (Love et al., 2001) also found that fear of offending the patient was an important screening barrier. A survey of a convenience sample of physicians and nurses working in emergency and urgent care departments found a variant of the patient offense barrier–fear of overstepping boundaries and intruding into private family matters (McGrath, Bettacchi, Duffy, Peipert, Becker, & St. Angelo, 1997).

In addition to research cited above suggesting that female patients approve of being asked by their health care providers about domestic violence, Hamberger, Ambuel, Marbella, and Donze (1998) found that battered women want their physicians to ask about domestic violence. Further, among primary care patients not selected for domestic violence, 78% reported favoring routine health care provider inquiry about domestic violence (Friedman et al., 1992). Health care providers routinely ask patients about a wide range of sensitive and "personal" issues such as range of sexual practices, sexual orientation, and so on. Therefore, when such questions are couched within other questions related to prevention and safety, presented in a matter-of-fact manner, there is little reason to believe that most patients will be offended. However, there are few studies that have evaluated the manner in which abuse screening questions can be asked in a minimally offensive manner. Brown, Lent, Schmidt, and Sas (2000) found that battered women were less comfortable with questions directly related to abuse than were nonbattered women. The researchers provided no evidence that battered women were actually offended by the questions about abuse. However, the latter study suggests that certain forms of questioning may facilitate patient comfort, and thus disclosure.

Perceived Time Pressures. Health care providers frequently cite time pressure as a major barrier to screening and helping partner violence victims. In focus groups with health care providers to identify barriers to screening, Minsky, Pape, and Hamberger (2000) report that many health care providers discussed feeling overworked and overwhelmed with their current staffing responsibilities and patterns. They viewed adding domestic violence screening and intervention as a major impediment to performing their other duties in a positive and professional manner. Providers frequently asked how they could possibly complete all of their duties within set timeframes when more requirements are added on to their list of duties. More indirect expressions of time pressure centered upon concerns about tying up rooms needed to maintain patient flow while providers worked with patients who admitted to abuse. A number of other researchers also identified the problem of time pressures interfering with domestic violence screening (Brown, Lent, & Sas, 1993; Ferris, 1994; Sugg, this volume; Sugg & Inui, 1992). Ferris' (1994) national survey of Canadian primary care physicians revealed that almost half (47%) listed time concerns as a major barrier, along with 40% of obstetrician-gynecologists (Parsons et al., 1995).

Perceived Irrelevance of Domestic Violence to Healthcare Practice. Despite efforts to persuade healthcare providers that domestic violence is a legitimate and important health care issue, many providers view it as outside the purview of their work (Fletcher, 1994). Minsky et al. (2000) found that many nurses reported failing to understand or accept responsibility for domestic violence. One respondent summed up this position in the following way: "How much responsibility do I own to save the world?"

A variation of the attitude that domestic violence is not relevant to medical or nursing practice is the notion that domestic violence screening is relevant, but not to the particular medical specialty and setting in which the respondent works. Minsky et al. (2000) found that staff working in Labor and Delivery strongly endorsed the notion that domestic violence posed significant dangers to both the mother and child to be born. However, they also opined that screening for domestic violence should have occurred during prenatal visits. They expressed concern that because their patients were primarily in active labor, screening was irrelevant to their immediate tasks of facilitating delivery. Similarly, emergency department staff expressed concern about the relevance of universal screening and found it improbable to screen patients for domestic violence who were seeking emergency services for conditions such as possible heart attack, stroke, or other potentially catastrophic illness (Minsky et al., 2000). Instead, staff in such departments preferred to screen in those situations in which their patients presented some clinical evidence of being in a violent relationship, such as suspicious injury pattern or depressed mood.

Support for such health care provider concerns is provided by women who were interviewed by McNutt, Carlson, Gagen, and Winterbauer (1999) about screening preferences in primary care settings. Ninety percent of respondents thought questions about domestic violence are appropriate when a patient presented for treatment of injuries, 62% and 71% believed screening questions were appropriate during gynecologic and obstetrical appointments, respectively; however, only 20% of respondents thought it was appropriate to ask about domestic violence when patients seek care for illness such as the flu. Hence, there may be types of appointments or patient presentations that are more appropriate screening venues. These appear to be extended visits for in-depth, health maintenance examinations. Symptom-focused visits for acute illness such as flu, and brief office visits for suture removal or blood pressure checks may not lend themselves to screening for domestic violence.

Although some researchers did not specifically identify perceived relevance among their study samples, comments related to time constraints suggested questions about relevance of screening, especially among practitioners who viewed domestic violence as rare (Moore et al., 1998; Parsons et al., 1995). Hence, the above review suggests that perceived relevance may be related to two different issues. One group of studies (Moore et al., 1998; Parsons et al., 1995; Sugg & Inui, 1992) suggests that perceived irrelevance of screening is related to false notions about the prevalence of domestic violence among a respondent's patient population. Minsky et al. (2000) also suggest that competing job demands and priorities may affect a clinician's belief about the relevance of domestic violence screening to their practice.

Fear of Loss of Control of the Provider-Patient Relationship. Family physicians and obstetricians/gynecologists have discussed their sense of powerlessness to "treat," "fix," or effectively help partner violence victims (Brown et al., 1993; Ferris, 1994; Parsons et al., 1995). Sugg and Inui (1992) found that primary care physicians frequently did not screen for domestic violence due to fear that once domestic violence was identified, it would set off a chain of events within the patient encounter that would wrest control of the entire encounter from the physician. Included in this "Pandora's Box" are strong emotional responses of the patient, time spent in crisis management, loss of control over the rest of the schedule, fear of litigation, fear of reprisal by the abusive spouse, and inability to control the outcome for the patient, to name a few. This fear of loss of control is important to health care providers, as evidenced by the high number of respondents in the Sugg and Inui study who mentioned it (42%).

Health care providers are accustomed to following protocols and treatment guidelines. They are trained to assess, diagnose, and prescribe treatment. Domestic violence does not lend itself so neatly to such a model (Warshaw, 1989). Working with domestic violence victims requires a collaboration that validates the victim's experiences and trusts that she makes decisions about her safety and survival that are rational and strategic, even if, to an outsider, they may appear otherwise. However, if control of the intervention process is the primary value, such collaboration cannot occur, and thus appropriate screening or intervention behaviors will not take place. In effect, Warshaw and others (e.g., Stark et al., 1979) hypothesize that effective medical management of domestic violence requires development and implementation of different models of patient care. To date, there is no research evidence comparing the relative effectiveness of different patient care models on screening and intervening into domestic violence.

Provider Attitudes and Accountability. Health care providers sometimes exhibit attitudes and behaviors that directly inhibit screening, identification, and help of abuse victims. For example, Loring and Smith (1994) concluded that health care providers both blame victims for the violence that happens to them, and hold them responsible for changing their situations on their own. Moore et al. (1998) found that some nurses held attitudes and beliefs about domestic violence that blamed the victim. Such beliefs include: (a) that some physical violence is to be expected in families, (b) there is no way to verify patient reports of abuse, (c) abuse is not a medical problem, and (d) abuse is none of the provider's business. Ferris (1994) and Rodriguez et al. (1999) identified physician victim blaming, including failure to screen because of the patient's failure to disclose abuse, and patient failure to follow-up with referrals and recommendations or end the violent relationship. Battered women reported to Hamberger et al. (1998) about a small, but palpable percentage of physicians who joked about domestic violence, asked patients what they did to trigger abuse, and encouraged the victim to go home and make up with her partner. In addition to the tremendous insensitivity exhibited by such behaviors, they blame the victim for both the violence that occurred to them, and for not ending it.

Kurz (1990) observed that battered women in emergency departments were treated differently, depending on whether they appeared to be intoxicated, unconventional, or evasive as to the cause of their injuries. Emergency department staff provided less complete interventions to women with such "discrediting attributes" (p. 248), including no response to the domestic violence aspect of the case. Larkin, Hyman, Mathias, D'Amico, and MacLeod (1999) observed that women presenting for emergency care with psychiatric conditions were less likely to be screened than women without such conditions. Hence, health care providers may also possess certain biases about who battered victims are, and judgments about whether they share responsibility for their situations. However, research to date has not directly assessed specific attitudes beyond self-report check-lists or focus group discussions. No specific attitude surveys related to domestic violence, victim presentation, and areas of responsibility have been conducted.

Gerbert, Johnston, Caspers, Bleecker, Woods, and Rosenbaum (1996) assessed health care provider attitudes indirectly, through the eyes of patients. Barriers related to health care providers identified by patients seem to reflect provider attitudes such as being uninterested, uncaring, and uncomfortable with domestic violence, victim blaming, and intolerance for women remaining with abusers.

Too Close for Comfort. For a number of health care providers, the issue of domestic violence creates sufficient discomfort that they simply avoid dealing with it professionally, as much as possible (Sugg & Inui, 1992). Ambuel, Hamberger, and Lahti (1997) discussed two types of providers for whom the issue of domestic violence could be personally overwhelming. The first type is one who may have grown up in a violent home, or may be presently experiencing domestic violence. Although many individuals in this category are highly motivated to help others struggling with partner violence, Ambuel, Butler, Hamberger, Lawrence, and Guse (2003) identified 18% of medical students that were too distressed and depressed about their own experiences to feel confident or motivated to help others in similar situations. In their national survey of obstetrician-gynecologists, Parsons et al. (1995) identified 13.1% of respondents who considered their personal abuse history a barrier to screening patients for domestic violence. A second scenario in which domestic violence issues are too close for comfort may occur among those providers who have no history of family violence (Sugg & Inui, 1992). For these individuals, accounts of survivors are shocking and emotionally overwhelming. Sugg and Inui's respondents indicated that discovering domestic violence in their patients exposed them to their own vulnerability.

Danger to the Provider. Only two studies identified fears for one's personal safety as a barrier to asking about domestic violence. Brown et al. (1993) observed that two of four focus groups of family physicians discussed fear for their physical safety if the perpetrator learns that the physician has screened or helped the victim. McGrath et al. (1997) reported that a "majority" of staff (p. 299) reported feeling danger to their personal safety as a barrier to screening and helping battered women.

Patient Barriers

As noted previously, patients who struggle with intimate partner violence rarely volunteer such information to their health care providers (Plichta, Duncan, & Plichta, 1996). Although, as we see from the review above, health care providers create many barriers to screening and identification, patients also create barriers to their own identification. Major barriers experienced by patients include lack of trust of the health care provider, fear of retribution if the perpetrator learns of the disclosure, fear of loss of control over decision-making to the health care provider, a sense of futility that the provider can help, and the way in which the victim defines her intimate relationship.

Lack of Trust. Although women victims of violent crime in general, and victims of partner violence in particular, make significantly more visits for health care services (Bergman & Brismar, 1991; Koss, Koss, & Woodruff, 1991), they are not highly likely to volunteer to health care providers that they are in violent relationships. McNutt et al. (1999) found that, of a sample of battered women from both medical and urban domestic violence programs, only 19% reported having volunteered being battered to their health care provider. In addition, 20% reported that they actually denied being abused when asked. Gerbert et al. (1996) were informed that such nondisclosure and overt denial are frequently intentional and strategic. In particular, health care provider behaviors that appear uninterested or uncaring in their overall approach to the patient are perceived by abuse victims as not trustworthy. Further, health care providers who appear uncomfortable with sensitive topics or seem to lack understanding of victimization issues also stimulate defensiveness from victims. No research has specifically studied trust, per se. Rather, the construct is inferred from patient reluctance to report domestic violence. It may be, as will be illustrated below, that the construct of "trust" is an overarching one that includes several barriers. For example, patients do not trust that the information they disclose will be kept confidential, and thus fear of retribution inhibits disclosure.

Fear of Retribution. Patients also fear that disclosure of abuse issues to a health care provider can lead to a series of events that culminates in retribution by the abuser (Gielen et al., 2000; Rodriguez et al., 1999). In medical settings, this can occur when the health care provider asks about domestic violence when other family members, including young but verbal children or the possible perpetrator, are present. It can also occur when the well-meaning health care provider receives the information in private, but, without patient consent, confronts the abuser in an effort to be helpful. Among marriage and family therapists, Hansen, Harway, and Cervantes (1991) found a strong tendency to treat domestic violence as evidence of an underlying communication problem, with a preference to treat the couple, rather than work with the victim alone and confidentially. Hamberger et al. (1998) recorded accounts from battered women that health care providers violated confidentiality by providing "counseling" with the abusive partner without the victim's consent. One outcome of a breach of confidentiality is violence or some other type of retribution, such as forced withdrawal from the medical or psychotherapy practice.

Fear of Loss of Control. In addition to concerns about retribution, abuse victims express other concerns about loss of control over their lives and efforts to cope with the violence. In particular, abuse victims frequently fear that disclosure of abuse will result in pressure to leave the relationship, and lead down an inevitable path toward dissolution of the relationship and loss of partner (Rodrigeuz, Craig, Mooney, & Bauer, 1998). This, in turn, can lead to other negative, albeit unintended consequences such as increased physical danger. Other related fears include loss of financial support and decreased standard of living for the victim, as well as the perpetrator, particularly if the perpetrator is the primary wage earner (Brown et al., 1993; Rodriguez et al., 1998). Hence, unless the patient is given strong assurances that screening and possible disclosure will result in collaborative practice to plan for safety, and not prescriptions to leave the relationship, a victim is not likely to acknowledge abuse.

Another fear that many victims have related to risk of disclosure is the possibility that they will lose custody of their children (Gerbert et al., 1996; Rodriguez et al., 1998). This could happen in a number of ways. If the healthcare provider determines that the children in the home are also at risk, they may decide that they must report their concerns to child protective services, triggering an investigation and possible removal. Another way abuse victims could lose custody of their children is through custody suits brought following dissolution of the relationship. McNutt et al. (1999) identified a number of additional areas that battered women fear loss of control over, including calling police without the patient's permission, lecturing and moralizing, giving empty assurances and euphemisms, and providing no response to a patient's disclosure.

Sense of Futility. Domestic violence is a pattern of coercion and control that pervades every aspect of the lives of victims. They experience periods of intense physical and sexual violence. In between are nearly constant periods of various forms of psychological abuse and control. Over time, victims have attempted many approaches to ending the violence in their lives, including changing their own behavior to appease their abusive partner, fighting back, going to counseling for themselves and for the relationship, consulting clergy for spiritual support, calling the police, and reaching out to family and friends. Many times, they may have met with "failure." They discovered that whenever they changed their own behaviors, the batterer changed the standards and found another reason to batter. When they fought back, the victim was beaten even harder or, in some situations, arrested for "abusing" their partners and ordered to "anger management" (Hamberger & Potente, 1994). If they reached out to family or friends, they may have been repelled for not following, or going against, advice. In addition, the batterer may have threatened friends and family, intimidating them and rendering them not helpful. Efforts to seek spiritual help and support may have resulted in entreaties to pray harder, live the faith, and above all, keep the family together (Miles, 2000). Counseling may have resulted in diagnoses, medication, and labeling of the victim as mentally ill (Rosewater, 1987). Efforts to live independently may have met with failure because of financial constraints and lack of job readiness (Loring & Smith, 1994). Although battered women are often conceptualized as suffering from low self-esteem and "learned helplessness," the experiences they have may better be understood as a massive failure of the system to help them become free from violence. Following so many failures, it should not be surprising that, as patients in a medical setting, they would not disclose abuse. From such a perspective, to do so would be to risk raised hopes and more disappointment. Under such circumstances, the healthcare provider's concerns, though well intentioned, are viewed as lacking credibility because the victim/patient does not know how the provider can help (Brown et al., 1993; Loring & Smith, 1994).

The Nature of the Intimate Relationship. The context of the partner violence is also an important factor when considering why battered women do not always readily disclose abuse. Abuse victims frequently report that they love their abusive partner. They want the violence to end, not the relationship. Dutton and Painter (1993) have discussed this in terms of traumatic bonding. That is, shortly after a violent incident, there may be a strong desire to disclose and do other things that would end the relationship. However, the focus on the positive aspects may also relate to a tendency to deny and minimize the level of violence and abuse in the relationship. Traumatic bonding may constitute a barrier by mediating hope within the abuse victim that the perpetrator will change and stop being abusive (Loring & Smith, 1994). Hence, she is reluctant to disclose abuse, because she believes he will change. However, to date, there is no research to support these hypotheses among abused women in medical settings.

Lack of Knowledge of Helping Resources. Hamberger et al. (1998) reported from a survey of battered women that one of the most important interventions that health care providers can provide is information about local resources for helping them. McNutt et al. (1999) reported that 38% of participants wanted their clinicians to be informed about available local services, and to provide such information to patients. Brown et al. (1993) found that physicians viewed patients as frequently reluctant to disclose abuse because they did not know or understand how the physician could help them. In addition, physicians viewed reluctant patients as lacking social supports to assist them in efforts to live violence free lives. More research about patient knowledge of local or health system barriers is needed to assess the types of knowledge gaps and concerns such patients have.

Embarrassment and Humiliation. Many women who live in violent relationships feel embarrassed and humiliated by their experiences and may be reluctant to tell others, including potential helpers, in an effort to save face. Gerbert et al. (1996) and McNutt et al. (1999) reported that battered women cited feeling uncomfortable, embarrassed, and ashamed to discuss abuse with their physicians. In fact, McNutt et al. indicated that such reasons were more prevalent than reasons related to external factors.

A Problem of Expectations: What Providers and Patients Expect of Each Other

The above discussion of provider and patient barriers suggests that each party comes to the provider-patient encounter with unique sets of barriers that unilaterally interfere with the goal of providing and receiving quality health care. A patient may come to a clinical encounter perfectly willing to talk about domestic violence only to have a provider show indifference to other sensitive needs, thus leading to a decision to deny abuse. Conversely, a provider may compassionately and comfortably ask about and discuss domestic violence, but confront a strong defensive stance on the patient's part. Unfortunately, in both instances, the patient and provider may share many values about domestic violence that, if known, could facilitate effective intervention and healing. Providers and patients may also possess misconceptions about the other, which, when unexpressed, continue a pattern of mistrust, lack of screening, and nondisclosure. For example, both Rodriguez et al. (1999) and Ferris (1994), in large-scale surveys of primary care physicians, found that doctor-patient cultural difference was a barrier to screening and intervention. Hence, some barriers to screening, identifying, and helping battered victims could be as much a function of the interaction as characteristics within the individual players. Unfortunately, it is often not clear what is meant by "cultural differences" between providers and patients. Because patients and providers potentially emerge from many different cultural and racial backgrounds and traditions, research is necessary to clarify the impact and relationship of cultural issues from specific cultures on barriers to screening for domestic violence in medical settings.

Unclarified Expectations and Other Communication Problems. Gerbert, Abercrombie, Caspers, Love, and Bronstone (1999) described what they called the "dance of disclosure and identification" (p. 122). That is, battered women offer a range of disclosures, from overt disclosures to subtle hints to lies about their abuse. Their hopes range from being identified to fear that identification will lead to more violence. On the other hand, physician providers who are successful in this area use approaches ranging from direct questions to hinting and indirect inquiries that are made over time. As the patient/victim feels increasingly confident that their provider will maintain confidentiality and possess the skill to help, she becomes more likely to disclose abuse.

Provider-Patient Gender Differences. Gender differences between provider and patient may also create a barrier to screening and intervention. Larkin et al. (1999) found that while male and female emergency department nurses were equally likely to screen for domestic violence, male nurses identified significantly fewer abused women. The authors speculated that male nurses might have communicated discomfort with asking the screening question through nonverbal cues or intonation. Conversely, because heterosexual abused women's abusers are male, the patient/victim may have been reluctant to disclose to a male provider. Brown et al. (1993) reported that male physicians expressed reservations that women abused by men would be willing and comfortable disclosing abuse to them. Hayden et al. (1997) surveyed current and past victims and found that almost three-fourths indicated that they would prefer to disclose and discuss domestic violence with a woman. Ferris (1994) found that female physicians were more likely than males to refer a battered woman to a shelter. Male physicians were more likely to refer abused patients to an attorney. Female primary care physicians experienced greater identification with female abused patients, and thus experienced a greater sense of their own vulnerability to abuse than males (Sugg & Inui, 1992). Male physicians expressed a greater fear of offending patients and damaging the doctor-patient relationship through screening. Both male and female physicians showed concerns for their patients by screening and making referrals. The different, gender-based concerns and behaviors, however, may have affected the abused patients' expectations of and satisfaction with treatment from their physicians, as well as their satisfaction with the overall provider-patient encounter (Plichta et al., 1996).

System-Level Barriers

If our analysis ended with consideration of provider and patient barriers to screening, identifying, and helping victims of partner violence, the implications would be clear. We would develop educational interventions to teach providers about the facts of domestic violence so as to counteract false misconceptions and provide new, accurate knowledge. In addition, such interventions would address provider attitudes, and help them develop a professional orientation toward partner violence as a legitimate health care issue. Further, providers would learn specific screening, identification, and intervention skills that fit within their respective professional purview. That having been accomplished, we would expect to see massive increases in screening, identification, and intervention with abuse victims in medical settings.

Unfortunately, Waalen, Goodwin, Spitz, Petersen, and Saltzman (2000) found in their review that education alone is not related to increases in screening and detection rates. Other factors intrinsic to the organizational system may come to bear to inhibit or prevent effective screening and intervention. Early evidence of this proposition was reported by McLeer, Anwar, Herman, and Maquiling (1989). They reported that inclusion of a systematic protocol for identification of abuse in an emergency department increased detection rates from about 5% to 30%. However, the system subsequently discontinued the protocol, following which detection rates reverted to near baseline levels. Beyond the study of McLeer et al. (1989), the research on system-level barriers to screening and intervention with abuse victims in medical settings is relatively sparse.

Minsky et al. (2000) were also concerned that training alone had a minimal effect on provider behavior. Training showed significant increases in provider self-efficacy, professional orientation toward domestic violence as a health care issue, and knowledge and skill at screening and referring abused patients (Hamberger et al., in press). However, following training, an audit of patient records revealed great variability of screening across clinical departments. A subsequent qualitative study with focus groups from a number of departments that serve many women revealed a number of systemic barriers that inhibited or precluded screening and intervention, even among those who valued such tasks and services. A major systemic barrier identified by several departments was high workloads. Respondents consistently stated that, in an era of lower staff levels and sicker patients in hospital settings, there were fewer resources to screen and help partner violence victims. Kheder (2001; Kheder & VandenBosch, 2001) reported that 58% of respondents in a three-hospital system identified time as a major barrier. However, in one hospital that had previously developed a domestic violence intervention program, the number of respondents reporting time as a barrier was 34%, lower than prior studies, suggesting that experience with screening and intervention may alter the perception of time as a barrier. Since the parameters of time constraints and heavy workload have not been systematically studied, the impact on screening constitutes an important knowledge gap, particularly given their importance in the literature as barriers.

Minsky et al. (2000) found that another significant system-level barrier that neutralized the effectiveness of an educational intervention was lack of a referral network, or an on-site patient advocate, to help abused patients. Roberts, Lawrence, O'Toole, and Raphael (1997) also speculated that lack of one during key hours might have impeded screening and documentation.

Staff also identified insufficient physical space that offered privacy for screening and intervention, particularly in emergency settings (Minsky et al., 2000). Some respondents noted that, in emergency settings, triage was conducted in the waiting room. Some emergency department treatment rooms had only curtains as room dividers (Kheder, 2001; Kheder & VandenBosch, 2001).

A further aspect of privacy relates to the question of screening if the female patient is accompanied by young children to the examination room. Zink (2000) found mixed agreement among physicians, child development experts, and domestic violence experts on the question of screening in front of young children. There was almost complete agreement on the feasibility of screening in the presence of pre-verbal children (i.e., less than 2 years old). There was considerable disagreement, however, about screening in the presence of older children, even if initial screening is general, focusing more on conflicts, anger, and disagreements. Hence, in some settings, such as family practice or pediatric clinics where young children frequently accompany their mothers, such involvement constitutes an important system barrier.

Another system barrier identified was lack of a process to give providers feedback on patient outcomes. Providers expressed concern and consternation that they were operating in the dark, and without feedback about the adequacy of their interventions, and were reluctant to invest more time and effort into the activity (Minsky et al., 2000).

Other providers questioned whether universal screening was relevant for their particular work setting. For example, providers in obstetrics and women and infants departments reported struggling with the competing organizational philosophies of family centered care versus the need to perform screening and intervention functions in privacy, even from other family members. Further research is needed to clarify the impact of broad organizational philosophy on patient care practice, and how competing philosophies and priorities evolve and create barriers to screening and intervention for domestic violence.

Cohen, DeVos, and Newberger (1997) studied systemic barriers to identification and intervention in five separate communities. The communities represented a spectrum of population, racial, and ethnic diversity and number and type of health care institutions. Overall, none of the communities addressed family violence comprehensively, in terms of programs, clinical practice norms, and policies. Instead, programs that did exist were driven primarily by strongly committed champions. Therefore, program longevity was highly dependent on the champion's tenure at a given institution. Within health care institutions, highly involved professionals and champions were typically marginalized professionally. Further, the ability of institutions to adequately address family violence was significantly affected by providers' prejudicial attitudes toward victim and perpetrator groups. Further, access of family violence victims to health services were generally inadequate due to unwillingness of private institutions to serve such patients, low Medicaid participation rates by the institutions, underinsured or uninsured status of many other patients, and poor public transportation to health care systems. Hence, this study suggests that larger system-level barriers that go beyond provision of privacy or time to screen and intervene may operate to inhibit provision of care to abuse victims. Of particular interest was the marginalization experience of those professionals who were committed to screening and intervention with abused patients. This suggests that health care systems and departments may develop social norms with respect to domestic violence interventions that informally and formally punish those who would do the work. More research in this area is needed to identify such norms and practices, as well as interventions for addressing them.

Is the Total Environment Domestic Violence-Competent? There is little, if any data on the type of total environment that would communicate to abuse victims that a particular system or clinical setting is a safe place to disclose and receive help for domestic violence issues. As noted above, provider and clinic/system credibility will of necessity be developed and earned over time through numerous encounters between providers, allied staff, reception staff, and others whom the patient/victim encounters. Clinics that appear cold and uncaring about basic patient concerns for respect, privacy, and competent and compassionate health care may be viewed by victims as threatening to their safety should they disclose (Ambuel et al., 1997). In contrast, Hamberger et al. (1998) found that battered women's preferences for physician interactions with them were consistent with provision of compassionate, respectful, and humane health care. Components of such health care include asking questions, performing thorough histories, conducting sensitive and gentle physical examinations, documentation, and follow-up. However, there is no research on the impact of the presence of posters and resource pamphlets on patient willingness to disclose abuse. Further, there is no research on the impact and effectiveness of training all clinic staff, including receptionists, administrative assistants, nurses, medical assistants, and other allied health professionals and physicians about domestic violence. Hence, aspects of clinic environments that facilitate patient disclosure and intervention remain to be determined.

METHODOLOGICAL ISSUES IN RESEARCH ON BARRIERS TO SCREEN AND IDENTIFY ABUSE VICTIMS IN MEDICAL SETTINGS

Many barriers to screening and helping domestic violence victims in medical settings have been identified in a number of studies that have surveyed providers and patients, alike. However, the state of research in this area is best characterized as foundational and seminal. Methodological weaknesses preclude firm conclusions about the type and nature of barriers that inhibit effective and consistent screening for domestic violence in medical and mental health settings.

Qualitative Studies

Many studies of barriers relied on focus groups (Brown et al., 1993; Gerbert et al., 1999; Minsky et al., 2000; Rodriguez, Quiroga, & Bauer, 1996; Sugg & Inui, 1992) and in-depth, individual interviews (Cohen et al., 1997; Gerbert et al., 1996). Such approaches provide a richness and depth of information that cannot easily be captured from self-report surveys. They are flexible, and investigators can ask follow-up questions to certain responses to develop a deeper understanding of the respondent's observations and comments. However, qualitative research based on focus group data, while important in developing understanding and ideas for further research, also has limitations. First, participants are typically not randomly selected for participation and frequently are recruited because of their particular experience and views on a particular issue. Second, focus group and in-depth interview studies in this area have small sample sizes.

In qualitative studies, such intentional selection procedures enable researchers to highlight specific issues. This research provides a rich source of hypotheses for further study. However, small sample size, nonstandardized, reflexive methods of inquiry, and thematic analysis preclude generalization to the general population, or even beyond the specific setting in which the participants work. Such research provides important leads for further development of concepts and constructs, as well as hypotheses for further, systematic study with large, representative samples. At present, however, very few large-scale studies have been completed.

Large Sample, Representative Sample Surveys

Large sample, representative surveys are important because they survey large samples of key stakeholders in a random manner that provides confidence that participants are representative of all or most stakeholders in the particular group under study. Because different disciplines and specialties may experience different barriers (Minsky et al., 2000), results of such representative sample surveys are limited to the stakeholder group under study. Conclusions drawn from studies of family physicians may not generalize to obstetricians-gynecologists, and so on. Rodriguez et al. (1999) surveyed the practices and attitudes of "primary care physicians," and included family physicians, internists, and obstetricians-gynecologists. They also included work setting as a variable. Rodriguez et al. found significant screening differences between primary care specialties and work setting. Obstetrics-gynecologists and physicians working in public clinics reported the highest screening rates. Internists in private practice and physicians working in health maintenance organizations (HMOs) showed the lowest screening rates. Hence, more research needs to be conducted to determine barriers, attitudes, and practices with specific specialties and disciplines and work settings.

Another methodological issue related to large scale, representative sample surveys is participation rate. In a national random sample of dentists, Love et al. (2001) attained a response rate of 56%. Parsons et al. (1995) reported a response rate of 14.6% for a national survey of obstetricians-gynecologists. Ferris (1994) and Rodriguez et al. (1999) reported response rates of 61% and 69%, respectively. Although response rates for the latter two studies approach acceptable levels, clearly the low response rate reported by Parsons et al. and the mediocre response rate reported by Love et al. raise questions about self selection bias and the generalizability of survey results.

Only Gielen et al. (2000) reported a case-control study of women's attitudes about domestic violence screening and the potential impact of mandatory reporting. Case-control studies, however, provide information about whether perceived barriers are specific to abused women or women patients, in general. Because proponents of screening advocate for screening of all patients, it is important to assess the preferences, attitudes, and concerns of all women. Hence, case control studies are an important methodological advance in the field.

Survey Instruments

In general, it appears that most studies that used standardized, self-report survey instruments to assess provider barriers, attitudes, and practices reported fairly comprehensive procedures for survey development. In particular, lists of barriers to be studied have generally been gleaned from previous literature (Parsons et al., 1995; Rodriguez et al., 1999), and thus are not developed *de novo*. In addition, most studies collaborated with experts in domestic violence to develop items, determine item face validity and content validity, appropriateness, and clarity (Ferris, 1994; Parsons et al., 1995; Rodriguez et al., 1999). All of the studies using standardized surveys also reported pilot testing to determine item face validity.

Ferris (1994) and Rodriguez et al. (1999) used single-item lists of possible barriers to which participants responded. Parsons et al. (1995)

used single items to measure "minor" barriers. While single item measures may represent a good start for measuring attitudes and barriers, there are psychometric and methodological problems with such an approach that limit conclusions drawn from such studies. First, basic psychometric properties of validity and reliability of single-item indices are suspect. Further, although a particular item may have face validity (i.e., appear to measure what it purports to), construct validity remains to be determined. That is, does the item actually measure the purported underlying theoretical construct? For example, an oft-cited barrier noted above is lack of time to screen. However, it is unknown from the current research whether the concept of time relates to the provider's perception of time pressures, actual system-imposed workloads, or some combination of the two. Another frequently mentioned barrier reviewed above is the patient's failure to follow through on referrals. However, it is unclear whether it is the actual patient "failure" or the provider's lack of understanding of domestic violence dynamics, or the provider's negative attitudes toward abuse victims, generally. Without examining in greater depth the concepts and constructs related to supposed barriers beyond face validity, inappropriate or ineffective interventions could be proposed and developed. Hence, at present, an important knowledge gap in this area involves the validation and further clarification of barriers that have been identified during this seminal stage of research. The model described by Parsons et al. (1995) for measuring "major" barriers represents a good start for development of valid measures of barriers and provider attitudes. They developed multiple items for each construct. The next step in survey development would include analysis to determine the most valid and reliable items and further validation testing using multiple groups.

A related concern is that current research does not inform us about the mechanisms by which various barriers exert their screening-inhibiting effects. For example, several studies have identified provider gender as a potential barrier to screening and identification. However, there are various possible explanations for such observed differences. Sex differences may relate to different types of fears and concerns experienced by male and female providers (Sugg & Inui, 1992). Males appear to fear damaging the doctor-patient relationship if they ask about abuse, whereas female providers appear to wish to avoid acknowledging their own sense of vulnerability. Although battered women reported greater comfort disclosing abuse to female providers than to male providers, reasons for this difference may not be as obvious as they seem. While female abuse victims may generalize their fear and reluctance to include discomfort with male providers, it may be that male and female providers engage in different types of behaviors that differentially affect the comfort levels of abused women. Therefore, as with many issues in this area, more research is needed to identify mechanisms by which various barriers inhibit screening.

Racial/Ethnic Issues

Very little research was reported that examined barriers related to ethnic/cultural issues in any depth. Rodriguez et al. (1996) purposely developed focus groups of women from a number of distinct ethnic groups, but patterns of similarity and difference between groups were not reported. Rodriguez et al. (1999) reported that 56% of their physician respondents listed "cultural differences" as a barrier to screening, but provided no further elaboration. In their focus group study, Gerbert et al. (1999) observed that physicians discussed the importance of individualizing screening and assessment practices to accommodate patient cultural and language barriers. However, no studies were found that specifically studied racial and cultural differences in barriers to domestic violence screening and intervention. Such studies are important because of racial disparities in health care access (e.g., Cornelius, 1997; Grumbach, Vranizan, & Bindman, 1997), as well as other research from health care settings that suggests that women of color may have different experiences and preferences for treatment of domestic violence issues. Hamberger et al. (1998) found that African American women expressed some differences from Caucasian women in preference for physician behaviors. In general, African American women were less rejecting of physician expressions of concern about their partners' well-being, suggestions for couples counseling, and matter-of-fact communication styles than were Caucasian women. Because such differences were not expected, and were typically from single-item responses, firm conclusions about the meaning or validity of such findings cannot be made. Nevertheless, such findings serve as a reminder of the need to study racial/ethnic and cultural issues when attempting to identify barriers to screen and intervene with abuse victims in medical settings.

OVERCOMING BARRIERS

Although many barriers to screening, identification, and intervention with abuse victims in medical settings exist, there is emerging evidence that they can be effectively addressed with appropriate interventions. Areas of intervention include education about domestic violence and skill-building in screening and intervention techniques, use of protocols, administrative interventions such as performance reviews, and continuous quality improvement approaches and creating patient friendly clinic environments.

The Role of Education

Although, as noted above, education alone has not been shown to significantly affect health care provider screening and intervention behavior (Waalen et al., 2000), it does appear to be a necessary part of any initiative to screen, identify, and help partner violence victims. In fact, some studies have shown a number of positive effects of education.

In the area of domestic violence, early research on the effects of education focused on retrospective reports of education during training years or participation in domestic violence related continuing education. In general, retrospective reports of health care professionals of a history of prior domestic violence education is inconsistently related to self reports of current screening behavior (Carbonell, Chez, & Hassler, 1995; McGrath et al., 1997).

Krueger and Schafer (2000) found no differences between medical specialties, attending physician/resident physician status, or state of practice as a function of participation in domestic violence-related continuing medical education. Only physician sex was related to screening rate. Practices with female physicians were four times more likely to conduct domestic violence screening than all-male practices. These findings appear to cast doubt on the positive impact of CME for domestic violence on self-reported screening rates for domestic violence.

A number of studies have evaluated the direct impact of training on objective indices of screening such as chart audit for screening completion. Mandel and Marcotte (1983) did not find training to increase screening rates and abuse identification. However, training was related to fewer inappropriate medication prescriptions and increased inquiry about safety in the home. Other researchers have likewise failed to detect change in screening behaviors following domestic violence training (Roberts, Lawrence, O'Toole, & Raphael, 1997; Saunders & Kindy, 1993). However, positive benefits of training were noted in other areas. Roberts et al. reported significant, positive changes in provider knowledge and attitudes, and Saunders and Kindy (1993) found that female physicians who received education conducted more thorough histories and safety planning.

Another series of studies has shown, like Roberts et al. (1997), that education has a positive impact on provider self-efficacy to screen and provide appropriate intervention (Hamberger et al., 2004; Harwell, Casten, Armstrong, Dempsey, Coons, & Davis, 1998; Thompson et al., 2000). These studies suggest that a 3-6 hour training session can lead to increased knowledge of what and how to ask about partner violence, increased knowledge of local resources, and increased sense of skill at being able to manage patient encounters that involve partner violence issues. Moreover, some of the positive effects of training on these knowledge and attitude areas were shown to persist for up to six months (Hamberger et al., 2004; Harwell et al., 1998). Therefore, even though an educational program alone appears to have minimal impact on health care provider screening behavior, it does appear to have other important benefits that can prepare the provider to screen if other barriers are addressed.

Impact of Protocols

Implementing written protocols or prompts has been found to significantly increase documented rates of screening and intervention with abuse victims (Waalen et al., 2000). Waller, Hohenhaus, Shah, and Stern (1996) reported on efforts to develop and validate a screening and referral protocol for use in emergency departments. They reported on complete data for 114 of 595 eligible female patients seen during a two-week period, for a 19% response rate. The overall sensitivity for the protocol was 50%, and specificity was 95%. Waller et al. attribute some of the difficulty validating their protocol to poor attendance at mandatory training to introduce the protocol, as well as staff confusion about the data collection procedures. Moreover, Waller et al. also described structural/organizational changes within the emergency department that significantly altered productivity requirements that may have adversely impacted the data collection process.

Olson, Anctil, Fullerton, Brillman, Arbuckle, and Sklar (1996) found that adding a screening prompt to the patient's chart resulted in significant increases in documented screening. Olson et al. evaluated the cumulative effect of adding a standard question to the patient data sheet, "Is the patient a victim of domestic violence?" and subsequent education on recognition of domestic violence in an emergency department.

The education intervention was not related to significantly greater domestic violence recognition.

Patel, Hamberger, and Griffin (2001) conducted a study similar to that of Olson et al. (1996) with family practice resident physicians. Patel et al. studied the cumulative effect of education and the inclusion of a screening question on the History form in a family practice outpatient clinic, and found the documented rate of screening rose to 92%. Hence, it appears, from the two studies above, that inclusion of a prompt on the patient's chart reminding or guiding the clinician to ask about domestic violence results in higher levels of screening and domestic violence recognition than not having the prompt.

Fanslow, Norton, Robinson, and Spinola (1998) assessed the impact of a domestic violence protocol on increasing identification and care of acutely abused patients in an emergency department setting. The quasi- experimental design of the study compared the effects of education and protocol implementation at one community emergency department with another, comparison community based emergency department in the same community. Chart audit assessed interventions offered, as well as quality of documentation, using previously described and published criteria.

Overall prevalence of documented domestic violence was found to be 2.6%. The training hospital showed a significant increase in classification from suspected to confirmed domestic violence following protocol implementation. In contrast, the comparison emergency department did not, and even appeared to show less classification of probable domestic violence. Additionally, the intervention hospital showed a marginal increase ($p < .06$) in documentation, improving documenting the perpetrator's relationship to the victim, use of a body map, and circumstances of the assault. Finally, the intervention emergency department staff showed a highly significant increase in use of intervention strategies, whereas the comparison hospital did not.

However, the research of McLeer et al. (1989) and McGrath et al. (1997) caution that protocols alone, without education and appropriate institutional support to overcome barriers, do not result in increased screening and intervention. Specifically, McGrath et al. found that protocols for domestic violence screening and identification were in place in all of the institutions from which they recruited health care providers to study screening patterns and barriers. However, only 24% of participating physicians and 34% of nurses stated that they were aware of the protocol's existence in their departments. Hence, for protocols to be effective, health care providers must first be aware and knowledgeable of how to use them.

Covington, Dalton, Diehl, Wright, and Piner (1997) conducted in-depth interviews with maternal care coordinators to determine factors related to increased reporting with a systematic protocol. The providers noted the written protocol and data collection form, as well as asking direct, specific questions about abuse, were helpful. In addition, the providers noted the value of conducting multiple assessments across the pregnancy, as domestic violence that may not emerge until later in the pregnancy would be missed with one-shot inquiries.

Wiist and McFarlane (1999) conducted a quasi-experiment to test the integration of the Abuse Assessment Screen (AAS; McFarlane, Parker, Soeken, & Bullock, 1992) protocol into routine prenatal health care with pregnant women in three matched, public health clinics. Ninety-six percent of the participants were Latina. Two clinics served as the experimental sites, and the third served as the control site. The study sought to determine the effect of the protocol on getting the AAS on each medical chart, use of the AAS, detection of abuse, and referral of abuse. Results showed significant increases in all of the above variables 12 months following introduction of the protocol, and no change in the comparison clinic.

The research in this area is limited in a number of ways, precluding drawing firm conclusions about the impact and value of written protocols and chart prompts for increasing screening behavior and identification of abuse in medical settings. The lack of true experiments does not allow for decisive evaluation of the impact of protocols. Olson et al. (1996) and Patel et al. (2001) essentially used AB group designs, introducing one intervention, then another, and measuring results. In both evaluations, it appears that education does not add to increases in screening behavior observed for introduction of a chart prompt. However, neither study made direct comparisons of both interventions. Further, no counterbalancing of interventions (i.e., education–protocol, protocol–education) was done in either study. Although it would be difficult to randomly assign health care providers from within the same clinic or institutional setting to different experimental or control conditions, the study by Thompson et al. (2000) provides a model for conducting such an experiment. Specifically, randomized, nested group designs, which assign entire clinical settings to experimental or control conditions, can be implemented. Such designs can be particularly useful when assessing the impact of one or two variables, such as the impact of written protocols or chart prompts, which may be more subject to experimental control than less specific, more global types of interventions such as "education." Lack of experimental trials represents a clear methodological gap in the field.

Finally, the work of McLeer et al. (1989) and Waller et al. (1996) showed that larger, system-level barriers can inhibit the possible positive effects of protocols. These studies serve as reminders of the difficulties in applying research designs in applied, clinical settings.

Administrative Interventions

Few studies have examined administrative-level interventions to facilitate screening and intervention into domestic violence by health care providers. Such interventions could potentially address barriers identified above related to institutions providing feedback to clinicians about the adequacy of their efforts, creating the position of in-house advocate to facilitate referrals, and holding clinicians accountable for screening and intervening as part of their job descriptions.

One study found that formally incorporating screening rates into providers' job description and quarterly performance review significantly increased screening rates among nurses (Larkin, Rolniak, Hyman, MacLeod, & Savage, 2000). Overall, pre-intervention screening rates were determined to be 29.5%. Following intervention, average screening rate for the department was observed to be 72.8%.

A number of recent studies (Harwell et al., 1998; Pape, Minsky-Kelly, & Hamberger, 2001; Thompson et al., 2000) described a continuous quality improvement intervention that included setting screening rate goals, conducting regular, random chart audits, and providing feedback to clinical departments. For example, in Pape et al. departmental leadership agreed to screening goals of 100%. Department managers were provided with regular reports on departmental screening rates relative to established goals. Specialized in-service training was conducted. Administrative trouble-shooting also occurred within each department to address ongoing barriers and problems. For example, a bi-lingual battered women's advocate was identified as a key contact person at the local abuse shelter. In addition, an administrative decision was made to integrate the screening question into the nursing assessment forms to function as a prompt. The researchers found that the intervention resulted in significantly increased screening and referral rates. Specifically, pre-intervention screening rates were near zero. Over 18 months of ongoing administrative intervention as described above, screening rates increased, on average across departments, to 87%.

Creating Victim Friendly Clinical Environments

Though there is little specific research available on the topic, the literature suggests that victims and survivors are very observant of environmental cues that provide information about whether it is safe for them to disclose abuse (Gerbert et al., 1999). Bolin and Elliott (1996) studied the question of whether patients would respond to doctors wearing buttons that said "It's OK to talk to me about family violence and abuse." The doctors who wore the buttons were trained to address domestic violence issues with their patients. Another group of doctors, also trained in domestic violence were randomly assigned to the "no button" condition. Physicians in both groups were trained to monitor and document conversations about domestic violence each day. Results showed significantly more discussion about domestic violence with patients among doctors wearing the buttons than among doctors without buttons. These results were the same for comparisons of total conversations about domestic violence and for number of working days per month in which domestic violence was discussed. This study suggests that health care systems can create environments that communicate immediate and concrete messages that its providers understand domestic violence and are trained and prepared to help in various, appropriate ways and that patients will respond positively to such cues. The physicians were not blinded to the study, and there is no way to rule out the possibility that the physicians may have unwittingly prompted more discussion about domestic violence on the days they wore the buttons than on the days they did not. Nevertheless, the study does point to the possibility and feasibility of investigating the impact of fairly simple, but potentially fruitful interventions to increase patient disclosure and discussion of abuse issues.

Other ways clinic environments can communicate similar messages include stocking exam rooms and restrooms with posters and brochures about family violence, training all staff to be sensitive to partner violence, and training all direct service staff to screen and provide basic emotional support to anyone who discloses domestic violence. These interventions have yet to be evaluated.

Taken together, the collection of studies suggests that abused women have fairly clear ideas about what constitutes helpful and effective health care provider interventions when they disclose the fact of abuse in their lives. Specifically, battered women value respect for their autonomy and decision-making abilities. But they also value emotional support and validation of their experiences. Further, abused women value careful examinations of the violence history and injuries. More-over, they value inquiry about the safety of children in the home, and documentation of the abuse. This research has informed the develop-ment of health care provider training curricula (Ambuel et al., 1997; Hamberger & Ambuel, 1997), as well as patient intervention programs (Harwell et al., 1998; Thompson et al., 2000). However, to date, there are no studies that have evaluated the impact of such interventions on the lives of abuse victims who are identified in medical settings. Minsky et al. (2000), Thompson et al. (2000), and Harwell et al. (1998) reported on increased screening rates, as well as increased rates of referral to a program for abused women. However, no data has been presented that documents how such interventions actually affect abused women. Questions to be answered in this area include whether the woman feels safer in her home, if she has a more comprehensive idea about commu-nity resources for safety, and whether she has a safety plan to increase the probability of escape or avoidance of abuse. In addition, it remains to be determined how and whether such interventions affect the health status of abused women, including mental and physical health indices, as well as perceived health status and health care utilization. Hence, the impact of health care interventions with abused women remains one of the major frontiers of research in this area.

Summary and Clinical Implications

As noted previously, health care providers who have direct responsi-bility for patient care have numerous opportunities to screen, identify, and help survivors and victims of partner violence. In addition, both health care providers and patients alike agree that domestic violence is an important health care issue and that health care can add to its amelio-ration. Despite such opportunities, however, the pattern and level of such screening has been found to be inconsistent and far from universal. In response to this disconnect between opportunity and practice, re-search have begun to investigate barriers that impede successful execu-tion of screening and intervention efforts. The result has been the identification and preliminary elucidation of barriers on a number of levels of the provider-patient, health care delivery process. Health care provider barriers include lack of knowledge of domestic violence and skill in asking screening questions and carrying out interventions that are helpful and safe. In addition, health care providers sometimes are ei-ther unaware of domestic violence as a health care problem or view it as irrelevant to their own practice settings, and thus not part of their professional responsibilities. Further, some health care providers are uncomfortable with the prospect of discussing partner violence with their patients. Areas of discomfort include feeling vulnerable or overwhelmed by the issue, either as a result of personal experience or due to the explosion of personal, closely held beliefs about the nature if intimate relationships. Still other discomfort may arise from fear of offending patients by asking about partner violence, and the possibility of losing control of the provider-patient encounter should screening result in a positive response. Perceptions of time pressures and heavy workloads besieged by yet another set of demands to take time to screen and help battered victims constitute yet another barrier faced by health care providers.

Even though battered women frequently respond to surveys in ways indicating that they value being asked by health care providers about domestic violence, as patients, they, too, face many barriers to acknowledging the violence in their lives. Like health care providers, battered women patients fear losing control of the provider-patient relationship and being swept into a system that is not of their choosing through mandated reporting, medication prescription, and advice to end a relationship before they are ready. Related fears center around concerns that the provider will violate confidentiality and confront the abuser, leading to further violence and isolation. Many such patients have learned that they cannot automatically trust their health care provider to have the knowledge, skill, or attitudes to respond therapeutically to any acknowledgement of violence, and hence may engage in a dance of disclosure whereby initial inquiries are met with denials, and only gradual admissions of problems and actual abuse. Finally, many battered patients feel shame, humiliation, and embarrassment at being abused, and are reluctant to admit it in response to a screening question.

Barriers to screening and intervention have also been located in the health systems in which providers work and patients seek help. These include lack of physical space to provide screening in a private, confidential manner, system-imposed workloads, and productivity demands. Systems can also contribute to lack of partner violence screening through failure to develop and specify appropriate referral networks and onsite advocacy. In addition, failure to give health care providers feedback on the adequacy of their screening rates and outcomes, as well as giving them direction on how to proceed with screening and intervention across departments and settings, also appears to impede screening and intervention.

Clinical Implications. Research on screening and intervention barriers is still in a fairly preliminary stage. Future research will need to continue to refine many of the concepts and develop measurement instruments that possess acceptable psychometric properties of reliability and validity. In addition, sampling will need to go beyond limited, intentional methods for hypothesis development to those that are more representative and generalizable. Despite limitations of the current literature, we believe it provides several important implications for providers and health system administrators for overcoming barriers to screening and helping partner violence victims and survivors.

First, although education about domestic violence has not been shown to be sufficient to increase screening behaviors, it is nevertheless indispensable to enable health care providers to develop appropriate attitudes and self-efficacy to effectively screen and help partner violence victims. Education can directly impact on several of the health care provider barriers described and discussed in this paper. Although optimal content of such education is yet to be empirically determined, it seems desirable to provide information on definitions of partner violence, as well as incidence and prevalence rates for particular health care settings, health impact, and dynamics of partner violence. Principles of screening and intervention that emphasize a collaborative care practice and respect for patient autonomy should also be included. Finally, to increase provider self-efficacy, they should be given opportunity to practice screening and intervention across a number of provider-patient scenarios. Ambuel et al. (1997) describe a detailed, model curriculum for screening and helping abuse victims, including prototypical questions for asking about both current and past partner and other forms of family violence.

Health care systems can help overcome patient barriers by providing patient-friendly environments that communicate system and provider sensitivity to and knowledge about intimate partner violence. Such an environment makes posters and pamphlets about domestic violence resources readily visible and available throughout the clinic setting, such as the waiting room, exam rooms, and restrooms. From their 20 years of experience, Thompson, Taplin, McAfee, Mandelson, and Smith (1995) note that posters and pamphlets placed in waiting rooms, rest rooms, and exam rooms can be a venue for "giving permission" to patients to discuss sensitive matters such as domestic violence. In addition, health care professional and allied staff are trained to understand partner violence and to respond to patients in a sensitive, caring manner. Not only should direct health service providers such as nurses, physicians, and social workers be educated about intimate partner violence, but all personnel who interact with patients in any way should receive at least basic education so that patient concerns are responded to nonjudgmentally, with respect for patient autonomy and well-being. These efforts may serve to enhance patient trust and confidence in the health system and its providers to effectively manage partner violence, as well.

Although education is a necessary component for reducing provider barriers it appears that education must be provided as part of a comprehensive, system-wide initiative to respond effectively to partner violence as a health care issue. Therefore, education programs may have to be tailored to the unique challenges faced by providers working in different settings. Further, a comprehensive program to screen and help battered patients will involve a multi-layered, multidisciplinary approach that goes well beyond a 1 to 3-hour lecture and seminar. A comprehensive approach, such as that described by Harwell et al. (1998) and Thompson et al. (2000) includes development of system-wide policies and procedures, screening and intervention protocols, and development of appropriate referral networks and resources for assisting victimized patients. In addition, the system must provide adequate space and privacy for conducting screening and protecting the confidentiality of patient disclosures.

Finally, health systems can develop and implement continuous quality assurance methods for assessing rates of screening, intervention, and referral of battered patients. Such methods provide important feedback to health care providers about the impact of their efforts and also function to enhance provider accountability for screening and associated clinical activities. In a related vein, continuous quality improvement efforts can lead to assessment and evaluation of the necessary components of intervention, as well as assess the impact of interventions on the quality of health and life of the affected patients.

At least one study (McCaw, Berman, Syme, & Hunkeler, 2001) sought to obtain outcome data following intervention (screening) for domestic violence. McCaw et al. successfully applied suggestions made by Thompson et al. (1995) regarding implementing a preventive program. These included establishing an environment that is supportive of the process, ongoing training of health care professionals, promoting enabling factors such as clear guidelines, reminders (i.e., posters in patient rooms), organized follow-up (i.e., data base), community alliances, and, very importantly, physician feedback regarding screening interventions.

During the study period the number of domestic violence referrals doubled. This was felt to be the result of providing an environment that supported domestic violence screening, training for primary care (emergency physicians and primary care physicians), as well as for specialty services (orthopaedic surgery, surgery, occupational medicine, and ophthalmology). Also, providing opportunities for patient self-referral through posters, pamphlets, and on-site access to community domestic violence resources was believed to have had a positive impact. Interestingly, patient awareness of domestic violence interventions and satisfaction also increased as the result of this research. The authors state that the ultimate goal of this research is to determine the health benefits that patients might realize from this intervention.

Research needs to continue in various areas of health care screening, including investigating aspects of clinic environments that facilitate patient disclosure and intervention, attempting to develop interdisciplinary consensus of clinical approaches to screening for domestic violence, investigating the costs and benefits of intervening with battered women in health care settings, and outcome studies on prevention efforts. Research that helps health care professionals identify victims readily and in large numbers, and provide appropriate interventions, has the potential to substantially impact the public health problem of domestic violence.

REFERENCES

Abbott, J., Johnson, R., Koziol-McLain, J., & Lowenstein, S. R. (1995). Domestic violence against women. Incidence and prevalence in an emergency department population. *Journal of the American Medical Association, 273,* 1763-1767.

Ambuel, B., Butler, D., Hamberger, L. K., Lawrence, S., & Guse, C. E. (2003). Female and male medical students' exposure to violence: Impact on well-being and perceived capacity to help battered women. *Journal of Comparative Family Studies, 34,* 113-135.

Ambuel, B., Hamberger, L. K., & Lahti, J. L. (1997). The family peace project: A model for training health care professionals to identify, treat and prevent partner violence. In L. K. Hamberger, S. Burge, A. Graham, & A. Costa (Eds.), *Violence issues for health care educators and providers* (pp. 55-81). Binghamton, NY: The Haworth Press, Inc.

American Academy of Pediatrics Committee on Child Abuse and Neglect. (1998). The role of the pediatrician in recognizing and intervening on behalf of abused women. *Pediatrics, 101,* 1091-1092.

American College of Emergency Physicians. (1995). Emergency medicine and domestic violence. *Annals of Emergency Medicine, 25,* 442-443.

American College of Obstetricians and Gynecologists. (1989). *The battered woman.* Washington, DC: American College of Obstetricians and Gynecologists.

American College of Obstetricians and Gynecologists. (2000). Domestic violence. *International Journal of Gynecology & Obstetrics, 71,* 79-87.

American Medical Association. (1992). American Medical Association diagnostic and treatment guidelines on domestic violence. *Archives of Family Medicine, 1,* 39-47.

Bergman, B., & Brismar, B. (1991). A 5-year follow-up study of 117 battered women. *American Journal of Public Health, 81,* 1486-1488.

Bolin, L., & Elliot, B. (1996). Physician detection of family violence. Do buttons worn by doctors generate conversations about domestic abuse? *Minnesota Medicine, 79,* 42-45.

Brown, J. B., Lent, B., & Sas, G. (1993). Identifying and treating wife abuse. *The Journal of Family Practice, 36,* 185-191.

Brown, J. B., Lent, B., Schmidt, G., & Sas, G. (2000). Application of the woman abuse screening tool (WAST) and WAST-short in the family practice setting. *The Journal of Family Practice, 49,* 896-903.

Burge, S. K. (1989). Violence against women as a health care issue. *Family Medicine, 21,* 368-373.

Carbonell, J. L., Chez, R. A., & Hassler, R. S. (1995). Florida physician and nurse education and practice related to domestic violence. *Women's Health Issues, 5,* 203-207.

Cascardi, M., Langhinrichsen, J., & Vivian, D. (1992). Marital aggression. Impact, injury, and health correlates for husbands and wives. *Archives of Internal Medicine, 152,* 1178-1184.

Clark, K.A., Martin, S. L., Petersen, R., Cloutier, S., Covington, D., Buescher, P. et al. (2000). Who gets screened during pregnancy for partner violence? *Archives of Family Medicine, 9,* 1093-1099.

Coben, J. H., Forjuoh, S. N., & Gondolf, E. W. (1999). Injuries and health care use in women with partners in batterer intervention programs. *Journal of Family Violence, 14,* 83-93.

Cohen, S., DeVos, E., & Newberger, E. (1997). Barriers to physician identification and treatment of family violence: Lessons from five communities. *Academic Medicine, 72*(Suppl.), 19-25.

Coleman, J. U., & Stith, S. M. (1997). Nursing student's attitudes toward victims of domestic violence as predicted by selected individual and relationship variables. *Journal of Family Violence, 12,* 113-137.

Cornelius, L. J. (1997). The degree of usual provider continuity for African and Latino Americans. *Journal of Health Care for the Poor and Underserved, 8,* 170-185.

Covington, D. L., Dalton, V. K., Diehl, S. J., Wright, B. D., & Piner, M. H. (1997). Improving detection of violence among pregnant adolescents. *Journal of Adolescent Health, 21,* 18-24.

Crowell, N. A., & Burgess, A. W. (Eds.) (1996). *Understanding violence against women.* Washington, DC: National Academy Press.

Dutton, D. G., & Painter, S. L. (1993). Emotional attachments in abusive relationships: A test of traumatic bonding theory. *Violence and Victims, 8,* 105-120.

Eastel, P. W., & Eastel, S. (1992). Attitudes and practices of doctors toward spouse assault victims: An Australian study. *Violence and Victims, 7,* 217-228.

Fanslow, J. L., Norton, R. N., Robinson, E. M., & Spinola, C. G. (1998). Outcome evaluation of an emergency department protocol of care on partner abuse. *Australian and New Zealand Journal of Public Health, 22,* 598-603.

Ferris, L. E. (1994). Canadian family physicians' and general practitioners' perceptions of their effectiveness in identifying and treating wife abuse. *Medical Care,* 1163-1172.

Fletcher, J. L. (1994). "Medicalization" of America: Physician heal thy society? *American Family Physician, 49,* 1995.

Friedman, L. S., Samet, J. H., Roberts, M. S., Hudlin, M., & Hans, P. (1992). Inquiry about victimization experiences. *Archives of Internal Medicine, 152,* 1186-1190.

Gerbert, B., Abercrombie, P., Caspers, N., Love, C., & Bronstone, A. (1999). How health care providers help battered women: The survivor's perspective. *Women & Health, 29,* 115-135.

Gerbert, B., Johnston, K., Caspers, N., Bleecker, T., Woods, A., & Rosenbaum, A. (1996). Experiences of battered women in health care settings: A qualitative study. *Women and Health, 24,* 1-17.

Gielen, A. C., O'Campo, P. J., Campbell, J. C., Schollenberger, J., Woods, A. B., Jones, A. S. et al. (2000). Women's opinions about domestic violence screening and mandatory reporting. *American Journal of Preventive Medicine, 19,* 279-291.

Grumbach, K., Vranizan, K., & Bindman, A.B. (1997). Physician supply and access to care in urban communities. *Health Affairs, 16,* 71-86.

Hamberger, L. K., & Ambuel, B. (1997). Training psychology students and professors to recognize and intervene into partner violence: Borrowing a page from medicine. *Psychotherapy, 34,* 375-385.

Hamberger, L. K., Ambuel, B., Marbella, A., & Donze, J. (1998). Physician interaction with battered women. The women's perspective. *Archives of Family Medicine, 7,* 575-582.

Hamberger, L. K., Guse, C. Boerger, J. Minsky, D., Pape, D., & Folsom, C. (2004). Evaluation of a healthcare provider training program to identify and help partner violence victims. *Journal of Family Violence, 19,* 1-110.

Hamberger, L. K., & Potente, T. (1994). Counseling women arrested for domestic violence: Implications for theory and practice. *Violence and Victims, 9,* 125-137.

Hamberger, L. K., Saunders, D. G., & Hovey, M. (1992). Prevalence of domestic violence in community practice and rate of physician inquiry. *Family Medicine, 24,* 283-287.

Hansen, M., Harway, M., & Cervantes, N. (1991). Therapists' perceptions of severity in cases of family violence. *Violence and Victims, 6,* 225-235.

Harwell, T. S., Casten, R. J., Armstrong, K. A., Dempsey, S., Coons, H. L., & Davis, M. (1998). Results of a domestic violence training program offered to the staff of urban community health centers. *American Journal of Preventive Medicine, 15,* 235-242.

Hayden, S. R., Barton, E. D., & Hayden, M. (1997). Domestic violence in the emergency department: How do women prefer to disclose and discuss the issues? *The Journal of Emergency Medicine, 15,* 447-451.

Hendricks-Matthews, M. K. (1991). A survey on violence education: A report of the STFM Violence Education Task Force. *Family Medicine, 23,* 194-197.

Hillard, P. J. (1985). Physical abuse in pregnancy. *Obstetrics & Gynecology, 66,* 185-190.

Hyman, A., Schillinger, D., & Lo, B. (1995). Laws mandating reporting of domestic violence. Do they promote patient well-being? *Journal of the American Medical Association, 273,* 1781-1787.

Kheder, S. (2001). Intimate partner violence: A health system's response–Part 2. *Continuum: (Society for Social Work Leadership in Health Care), 21,* 10-15.

Kheder, S., & VandenBosch, T. (2001). Intimate partner violence: A health system's response. *Continuum (Society for Social Work Leadership in Health Care), 21,* 15-22.

Koop, C. E., & Lundberg, G. D. (1992). Violence in America: A public health emergency. *Journal of the American Medical Association, 267,* 3075-3076.

Koss, M. P., Koss, P. G., & Woodruff, W. J. (1991). Deleterious effects of criminal victimization on women's health and medical utilization. *Archives of Internal Medicine, 151,* 342-347.

Krueger, P. M., & Schafer, S. (2000). Physician awareness of domestic violence: Does continuing medical education have an impact? *Journal of the American Osteopathic Association, 100,* 145-148.

Kurz, D. (1990). Interventions with battered women in health care settings. *Violence and Victims, 5,* 243-256.

Larkin, G. L., Hyman, K. B., Mathias, S. R., D'Amico, F., & MacLeod, B. A. (1999). Universal screening for intimate partner violence in the emergency department: Importance of patient and provider factors. *Annals of Emergency Medicine, 33,* 669-675.

Larkin, G. L., Rolniak, S., Hyman, K. B., MacLeod, B. A., & Savage, R. (2000). Effect of an administrative intervention on rates of screening for domestic violence in an urban emergency department. *American Journal of Public Health, 90,* 1444-1448.

Loring, M. T., & Smith, R. W. (1994). Health care barriers and interventions for battered women. *Public Health Reports, 109,* 328-338.

Love, C., Gerbert, B., Caspers, N., Bronstone, A., Perry, D., & Bird, W. (2001). Dentists' attitudes and behaviors regarding domestic violence. The need for an effective response. *Journal of the American Dental Association, 132,* 85-93.

Mandel, J. B., & Marcotte, D. B. (1983). Teaching family practice residents to identify and treat battered women. *Journal of Family Practice, 17,* 708-716.

McCaw, B., Berman, W. H., Syme, S. L., & Hunkeler, E. F. (2001). Beyond screening for domestic violence. A systems model approach in a managed care setting. *American Journal of Preventive Medicine, 21,* 170-176.

McFarlane, J., Parker, B., Soeken, K., & Bullock, L. (1992). Assessing for abuse during pregnancy. Severity and frequency of injuries and associated entry into prenatal care. *Journal of the American Medical Association, 267,* 3176-3178.

McGrath, M. E., Bettachi, A., Duffy, S. J., Peipert, J. F., Becker, B. M., & St. Angelo, L. (1997). Violence against women: Provider barriers to intervention in emergency departments. *Academic Emergency Medicine, 4,* 297-300.

McGrath, M. E., Hogan, J. W., & Piepert, J. F. (1998). A prevalence survey of abuse and screening for abuse in urgent care patients. *Obstetrics & Gynecology, 91*, 511-514.

McLeer, S. V., Anwar, R. A. H., Herman, S., & Maquiling, K. (1989). Education is not enough: A systems failure in protecting battered women. *Annals of Emergency Medicine, 18*, 651-653.

McNutt, L., Carlson, B. E., Gagen, D., & Winterbauer, N. (1999). Reproductive violence screening in primary care: Perspectives and experiences of patients and battered women. *Journal of the American Medical Women's Association, 54*, 85-90.

Miles, A. (2000). *Domestic violence. What every pastor needs to know.* Minneapolis, MN: Augsburg Fortress.

Minsky, D., Pape, D., & Hamberger, L.K. (2000, August). *Domestic violence: Qualitative analysis of barriers to identification and referral of victims in an urban healthcare setting.* Paper presented at the meeting of the American Psychological Association, Washington, DC.

Moore, M. L., Zaccaro, D., & Parsons, L. H. (1998). Attitudes and practices of registered nurses toward women who have experienced abuse/domestic violence. *Journal of Obstetrical and Gynecological Nursing Network, 27*, 175-182.

Novello, A. C. (1992). 'The hidden epidemic.' Physician leadership is essential. *Archives of Family Medicine, 1*, 29-31.

Olson, L., Anctil, C., Fullerton, L., Brillman, J., Arbuckle, J., & Sklar, D. (1996). Increasing emergency physician recognition of domestic violence. *Annals of Emergency Medicine, 27*, 741-746.

Pape, D., Minsky-Kelly, D., & Hamberger, L. K. (2001, September). *A long, bumpy, but worthwhile trip: Creating organizational change.* 11th Nursing Network on Violence Against Women International Conference, Madison, WI.

Parsons, L. H., Zaccaro, D., Wells, B., & Stovall, T. G. (1995). Methods of and attitudes toward screening obstetrics and gynecology patients for domestic violence. *American Journal of Obstetrics and Gynecology, 173*, 381-387.

Patel, D., Hamberger, L. K., & Griffin, E. (2001, September). *Additive impact of training and a written protocol for screening and documentation of domestic violence by family physicians.* Paper presented at the meeting of the Nursing Network on Violence Against Women International, Madison, WI.

Plichta, S. B., Duncan, M. M., & Plichta, L. (1996). Spouse abuse, patient-physician communication, and patient satisfaction. *American Journal of Preventive Medicine, 12*, 297-303.

Rath, G. D., Jarratt, L. G., & Leonardson, G. (1989). Rates of domestic violence against adult women by men partners. *Journal of the American Board of Family Practice, 2*, 227-233.

Roberts, G. L., Lawrence, J. M., O'Toole, B. I., & Raphael, B. (1997). Domestic violence in the emergency department: 2. Detection by doctors and nurses. *General Hospital Psychiatry, 19*, 12-15.

Rodriguez, M. A., Bauer, H. M., McLoughlin, E., & Grumbach, K. (1999). Screening and intervention for intimate partner abuse. Practices and attitudes of primary care physicians. *Journal of the American Medical Association, 282*, 468-474.

Rodriguez, M. A., Craig, A. M., Mooney, D. R., & Bauer, H. M. (1998). Patient attitudes about mandatory reporting of domestic violence. Implications for health care professionals. *Western Journal of Medicine, 169*, 337-341.

Rodriguez, M. A., Quiroga, S. S., & Bauer, H. M. (1996). Breaking the silence: Battered women's perspectives on medical care. *Archives of Family Medicine, 5,* 153-158.

Rosewater, L. B. (1987). The clinical and courtroom applications of battered women's personality assessments. In D. J. Sonkin (Ed.), *Domestic violence on trial: Psychological and legal dimensions of family violence* (pp. 86-95). New York: Springer.

Saunders, D. G., Hamberger, L. K., & Hovey, M. (1993). Indicators of woman abuse based on a chart review at a family practice center. *Archives of Family Medicine, 2,* 537-543.

Saunders, D. G., & Kindy, Jr., P. (1993). Predictors of physicians' responses to woman abuse: The role of gender, background and brief training. *Journal of General Internal Medicine, 8,* 606-609.

Stark, E., Flitcraft, A., & Frazier, W. (1979). Medicine and patriarchal violence: The social construction of a "private" event. *International Journal of Health Services, 9,* 461-493.

Sugg, N. (2006). What do medical providers need to successfully intervene with intimate partner violence? *Journal of Aggression, Maltreatment & Trauma, 12*(2/3), 103-123.

Sugg, N. K., & Inui, T. (1992). Primary care physician's response to domestic violence. Opening Pandora's box. *Journal of the American Medical Association, 267,* 3157-3160.

Surgeon General. (1985, October 27-29). *Surgeon General's workshop on violence and public health.* Leesburg, VA. Rockville, MD: Office of Maternal and Child Health, Bureau of Maternal and Child Health and Resources Development, Health and Human Services; 1986. Report to the Senate Committee on Children, Families, Drugs and Alcoholism.

Thompson, R. S., Rivara, F. P., Thompson, D. C., Barlow, W. E., Sugg, N. K., Maiuro, R. D. et al. (2000). Identification and management of domestic violence. A randomized trial. *American Journal of Preventive Medicine, 19,* 253-263.

Thompson, R. S., Taplin, S. H., McAfee, T. A., Mandelson, M. T., & Smith, A. E. (1995). Primary and secondary prevention services in clinical practice. Twenty years' experience in development, implementation, and evaluation. *Journal of the American Medical Association, 273,* 1130-1135.

Waalen, J., Goodwin, M. M., Spitz, A. M., Petersen, R., & Saltzman, L. E. (2000). Screening for intimate partner violence by health care providers. Barriers and interventions. *American Journal of Preventive Medicine, 19,* 230-237.

Waller, A. E., Hohenhaus, S. M., Shah, P. J., & Stern, E. A. (1996). Development and validation of an emergency department screening and referral protocol for victims of domestic violence. *Annals of Emergency Medicine, 27,* 754-760.

Warshaw, C. (1989). Limitations of the medical model in the care of battered women. *Gender and Society, 3,* 506-517.

Wiist, W. H., & McFarlane, J. (1999). The effectiveness of an abuse assessment protocol in public health prenatal clinics. *American Journal of Public Health, 89,* 1217-1221.

Wilt, S., & Olson, S. (1996). Prevalence of domestic violence in the United States. *Journal of the American Medical Women's Association, 51,* 77-82.

Zink, T. (2000). Should children be in the room when the mother is screened for partner violence? *The Journal of Family Practice, 49,* 130-136.

doi:10.1300/J146v13n03_04

What Do Medical Providers Need
to Successfully Intervene
with Intimate Partner Violence?

Nancy Sugg

SUMMARY. Increasingly, medical providers (physicians and mid-level providers) rely on research evidence to inform their medical practice. In order for medical providers to accept their role in diagnosing and intervening with IPV, they need clinical tools and institutional support. This paper explores the tools (prevalence rates, screening questions, intervention strategies) and support (educational, institutional, professional, research) needed to assist medical providers in successfully intervening with IPV. It also looks at the importance of guidelines and expert consensus panel statements to help establish best clinical practices when direct research evidence is lacking or conflicting. doi:10.1300/J146v13n03_05 *[Article copies available for a fee from The Haworth Document Delivery Service: 1-800-HAWORTH. E-mail address: <docdelivery@haworthpress.com> Website: <http://www.HaworthPress.com> © 2006 by The Haworth Press, Inc. All rights reserved.]*

KEYWORDS. Intimate partner violence, physicians, medical providers, intervention, research, evidence-based medicine

---

Address correspondence to Nancy Sugg, MD, MPH, Pioneer Square Clinic, 206 3rd Avenue South, Seattle, WA 98115 (E-mail: sugg@u.washington.edu).

[Haworth co-indexing entry note]: "What Do Medical Providers Need to Successfully Intervene with Intimate Partner Violence?" Sugg, Nancy. Co-published simultaneously in *Journal of Aggression, Maltreatment & Trauma* (The Haworth Maltreatment & Trauma Press, an imprint of The Haworth Press, Inc.) Vol. 13, No. 3/4, 2006, pp. 101-120; and: *Prevention of Intimate Partner Violence* (ed: Sandra M. Stith) The Haworth Maltreatment & Trauma Press, an imprint of The Haworth Press, Inc., 2006, pp. 101-120. Single or multiple copies of this article are available for a fee from The Haworth Document Delivery Service [1-800-HAWORTH, 9:00 a.m. - 5:00 p.m. (EST). E-mail address: docdelivery@haworthpress.com].

Evidence-based medicine is the watchword of the day in the medical world. Health care providers are demanding scientific proof of the efficacy of new treatments and interventions and a rigorous reappraisal of older therapies. No longer satisfied with continuing practices based on anecdotal evidence or historical entrenchment, and unwilling to squeeze unproven new interventions into already packed clinic agendas, providers look to published studies to guide and support their decisions. The gold standard of "proof" of efficacy is the randomized controlled trial. Randomized controlled trials, when well executed, provide important and accurate information, although by their very nature are often time consuming and expensive. Unfortunately, although the efficacies of drugs or surgical interventions are neatly studied by randomized control trials, other medical issues, such as intimate partner violence (IPV), do not lend themselves so readily. Conflicting definitions, small sample size or response rate, unreliable data due to the sensitive nature of the topic, and the myriad of biases innate to survey instruments hamper even the study of prevalence for IPV. This lack of traditional data leaves many health care providers wary of or resistant to incorporating IPV assessment and intervention into their practice.

So what do medical providers need in order to accept IPV as part of their professional purview and be successful in intervening? Initially, providers need evidence that domestic violence is prevalent in their specific clinic population. Next, a short, valid assessment tool and a succinct intervention with reliable and significant outcomes must be available. Finally, and probably most importantly, institutional support extending from the site of practice to professional medical associations must be in place to sustain the medical providers in continuing to intervene with domestic violence. Research plays a vital role in informing each of these above areas.

MOTIVATION

At the start, medical providers will question whether IPV is prevalent in their practice population. Fortunately, abundant research data exists documenting the significant number of patients experiencing domestic violence regardless of the practice setting. Data from primary care clinics (Fairchild, Fairchild, & Stoner, 1998; Gin, Ruker, Frayne, Cygan, & Hubbell, 1990; Hamberger, Saunders, & Hovey, 1992; Johnson & Elliott, 1997; McCauley et al., 1995; Rath, Jarrett, & Leonardson, 1989), although not amenable to direct comparison due to methodological differences, show substantial numbers of women currently or previously experiencing violence with intimate partners. The percentage of patients currently (within the past year) physically abused by an intimate partner ranged from 5.5% (McCauley et al., 1995) to 22.7% (Hamberger et al., 1992). Prevalence rates in primary care clearly indicate the extent of the problem. Turning to obstetrics, a specialty with a primary care overlay, studies find a significant rate of physical abuse during pregnancy. Comparing these multiple studies, Gazmararian, Lazorick, Spitz, Ballard, Saltzman, and Marks (1996) found a prevalence of violence during pregnancy ranging from 0.9% to 20.1%, with the majority of studies ranging 3.9% to 8.3%.

Literature can be found in a wide variety of specialties, including Gastroenterology (Drossman, Leserman, Nachman, Li, Gluck, & Toomey, 1990), ENT (Le, Dierks, Ueeck, Homer, & Potter, 1999; Perciaccante, Ochs, & Dodson, 1999; Zachariades, Koumoura, & Konsolaki-Agouridaki, 1990), Pain Center (Domino & Haber, 1987; Haber & Roos, 1985), Rehabilitation Medicine (Young, Nosek, Howland, Chanpong, & Rintala, 1997), and Ophthalmology (Beck, Freitag, & Singer, 1996), documenting the significant prevalence of intimate partner violence. The psychiatric literature offers multiple small studies drawn predominantly from inpatient psychiatric units or patients seeking marital counseling showing a significant rate of physical violence experienced by psychiatric patients (Cascardi, Langhinrichsen, & Vivian, 1992; Cascardi, Mueser, DeGiralomo, & Murrin, 1996; Jacobson & Richardson, 1987). Not surprisingly, the Emergency Department (ED) is a treatment site with a high prevalence of women seeking care for domestic violence related illness or injury. The high prevalence of current and/or lifetime physical assault by intimate partners is well documented by multiple ED studies (Abbott, Johnson, Koziol-McLain, & Lowenstein, 1995; Ernst, Weiss, Cham, & Marquez, 1997; Roberts, O'Toole, Raphael, Lawrence, & Ashby, 1996). Regardless of the practice site, domestic violence will be found in the population, and the literature is available to support this assertion.

Once medical providers are apprised of the evidence that DV exists in all patient populations, the next question is whether IPV is a medical problem. This change from perceiving IPV as a social, moral, economic, or psychological problem to acknowledging it as an active medical problem is often difficult for providers. Many relegate the care of patients affected by IPV to the realm of social work, lacking any working knowledge of the medical consequences of domestic violence. Fortunately, once again, abundant medical evidence supports domestic violence as well within the medical purview (Campbell et al., 2002). McCauley et al.'s 1995 study revealed that women experiencing domestic violence had more physical symptoms, scored higher for depression, anxiety, somatization, and were more likely to be abusing drugs or alcohol. In a gastroenterology clinic, Drossman et al. (1990) reported that abused women were more likely to have multiple somatic complaints, functional GI disorders, and lifetime history of surgeries. Danielson, Moffitt, Caspi, and Silva (1998) presented data from a birth cohort showing that over half the women victimized by an intimate partner had a DSM-III-R psychiatric diagnosis. Campbell and Lewandowski's 1997 review of the mental and physical health effects of IPV provides extensive documentation of the physical injuries, stress-related illnesses, infectious disease exposure, and increase risk of depression and PTSD. Clearly, IPV falls firmly in the medical purview due to the physical and emotional sequelae of abuse. Although multiple symptoms and illnesses have been statistically linked to IPV, there is no clear pathognomonic injury or symptom syndrome that can reliably be used to distinguish abused versus non-abused patients. Therefore, all women, and frankly all patients regardless of gender, need to be screened for IPV.

ASSESSMENT

The prevalence and medical consequences of domestic violence have been well established in the literature. The next important tool for medical providers is a short, valid, and reliable assessment instrument. The key word is short. Time limitations create real and unrelenting pressures on medical providers. Tools such as the 19-item Conflict Tactics Scale and the 30-item Index of Spouse Abuse are valuable in research but their length precludes their usefulness in the clinical setting. Several shorter instruments have been developed, often using the CTS and/or the ISA as the gold standard for comparison. The Abuse Assessment Screen (AAS; McFarlane, Soeken, & Wiist, 1992), HITS (Sherin, Sinacore, Li, Zitter, & Shakil, 1998), and Partner Violence Screen (PVS; Feldhaus, Koziol-McLain, Amsbury, Norton, Lowenstein, & Abbott, 1997) represent efforts to develop shorter reliable tools for use in a variety of clinical settings. However, even the shorter versions require asking 3 to 5 questions, which would be unacceptable for quick assessment in most practices. In addition to IPV, providers must also screen for HIV risk, CAD risk, alcohol, tobacco, and drug abuse, depression, and a variety of other health risks. The argument cannot be made with any credibility that IPV is more of a morbidity or mortality issue than the other health risks. If each health habit assessment required 3 to 5 questions, the providers would truly be overwhelmed in attempting to provide preventive medical care. More importantly, patients rarely present solely for preventive medical care. Acute and chronic medical problems must be addressed first, often leaving little time for health risk assessment. Given these limitations, if the goal is to assess all patients for IPV, regardless of risk factors, then a succinct tool of no more than two questions is required. Otherwise providers will not find the tool acceptable and it will not be widely used. The longer 3 to 5 question assessment tools are valuable for situations in which the clinical suspicion is high or the patient presents with significant risk factors.

Given the limitation of creating a 1- or 2-question assessment tool, what is being assessed must be clarified. Is the assessment for current abuse or any abuse past or present? The answer to this question will likely vary from one practice site to another. In the Emergency Department (ED), the questions will likely focus on current abuse. In primary care, any lifetime abuse would potentially have current medical consequences. If the central question is current abuse, what defines current: abuse directly resulting in the current visit, abuse within the past month, abuse during the current pregnancy, abuse within the past 6 months? The danger of an abusive episode is more than just the chronology of when it occurred. A recent episode of abuse that did not involve injury may be less dangerous than one occurring the previous month but resulting in significant injury. The questions must be framed to capture the time period of most interest for the particular medical setting.

Are the questions meant to assess all types of abuse (physical, sexual, and emotional) or only physical injury? Again, the focus will vary depending on the medical practice site. The importance of physical abuse is perhaps easiest for medical providers to acknowledge as it fits neatly with the concept of injury prevention. Providers do not need to make judgements regarding acceptable versus unacceptable behavior when the behavior in question can potentially cause injury. Direct questions about specific acts of physical violence (hit, slapped, pushed, etc.) can be formulated avoiding the more inflammatory wording of abused or battered or victim.

Questions regarding emotional abuse are much more difficult to formulate. What defines emotional abuse? Comments considered demeaning to one person might not be to another. Questions about emotional abuse stand a greater chance of appearing judgmental or paternalistic, increasing providers' discomfort in asking. Assessing for emotional abuse does not readily fit into one "yes/no" question, but requires exploring the effect of the verbal and emotional expressions of their partner on the patient's health and well being.

Inquiring into sexual abuse is fraught with similar difficulties. Culturally, a "norm" does not exist for acceptable sexual practices within the context of marriage or an intimate relationship. An act viewed as exciting and arousing to one person may be experienced as demeaning and abusive to another. The litmus test for defining abusive sexual acts is determining how these acts affect the emotional and physical well being of those involved. These questions are again not amenable to one "yes" or "no" answer. Furthermore, the concept of marital rape is very difficult for many people, including medical providers and patients, to fully grasp. The notions of "wifely duties" and "marital rights" for husbands are still prevalent in our society. The perception remains that by virtue of a marriage license, wives consent to performing sexual acts with their husbands, and are in fact obligated to do so. In reality, sex that is coerced or violently forced must be viewed as rape regardless of whether the perpetrator is a stranger or a husband. Non-consensual sex is as physically violent as hitting or punching, and due to the intimate nature of the acts is often more emotionally harmful. Needless to say, many medical providers are extremely uncomfortable asking patients about their sexual practices with spouses or partners. Similarly, patients often feel humiliated and distressed to reveal sexual abuse to their providers. Time and thoughtfully crafted questions are crucial to sensitively explore this area.

Learning to recognize the many types of IPV is an extremely important aspect of medical provider education. However, attempting to exhaustively assess for all possible forms of abuse is not possible in an initial assessment tool. It must be kept in mind that the initial assessment questions for medical screening are designed as a quick and efficient probe to determine if a disease process is present. The response to the probe questions will determine if further evaluation is indicated. An analogy is mammography. A screening mammogram is performed on an asymptomatic patient. If a suspicious lesion is found, then further diagnostic tests are ordered to determine the nature of the lesion. The same is true for IPV. The patient's answers to a short set of questions determine if further evaluation by a more in-depth set of questions is warranted. The more extensive questions will determine the diagnosis of IPV. An assessment tool that casts a wide net to capture all potential forms of abuse, but requires eight questions to administer, will not be utilized by medical providers. Researchers, clinicians, and advocates need to hone down to the essential elements of IPV relevant to a particular clinical site and determine if these elements are adaptable to as short, acceptable assessment tool.

The focus of assessment is often the primary recipient of interpersonal violence; as well, it should be given that this is the person at highest risk for illness, injury, and death. However, the crux of the problem of IPV is the perpetrator. In order to intervene with IPV, the assessment needs to encompass both recipients and perpetrators of abuse. Assessing for perpetrators gets at the root of the abuse and should be the ultimate goal. Furthermore, the dynamics of IPV do not always offer one perpetrator and one recipient of violence. In homes where IPV exists, the role of perpetrator or recipient can shift back and forth. The violence can be bi-directional, in one instance a patient can initiate the violence and at another time be the primary recipient. Although women are more likely to be injured by IPV, both women and men can be perpetrators and recipients, and both are at risk for the health consequences of abuse. Assessment tools that can screen for both recipients and perpetrators of violence will further the objective of decreasing IPV. Questioning the presence of any violence in the home will assist patients in examining the effect of violence on their health and safety, as well as the health and safety of their children.

Finally the assessment tool must be culturally appropriate. Culture must be understood in a broader sense than simply Caucasian, Afro-American, Asian, or Latino. Groups that share cultural norms must have assessment tools that are relevant to them. Teenagers, disabled persons, same sex partners, the elderly, and men are examples of groups that may require special adaptations to the questions used for assessment. Additional adaptations may be required for other groups such as hearing impaired, illiterate, or developmentally delayed.

Most importantly, the assessment tool must be valid. The tool must clearly measure IPV. Establishment of validity is very difficult lacking a gold standard for abuse. Abuse cannot be definitively diagnosed by a biopsy, blood test, or radiographic image. The diagnosis is based on the patient's oral history. Support for the history may be obtained from witnesses at the scene, police or ambulance reports, or injury patterns on exam. But ultimately, the diagnosis rests with the patient's account of the abusive behavior of their partner. Determining the validity and positive predictive value of an assessment tool is challenging given this limitation.

The above requirements make the development of an assessment tool appear formidable. Clearly, a variety of short assessment tools need to be formulated that respond to the needs of different patient populations and practice sites. A "one size fits all" approach will not work. And again, it needs to be kept in mind that the assessment tool is used to do an initial screening for IPV. A positive response to an assessment tool may then require further diagnostic questions to elucidate the nature and extent of the problem.

Once the tool is developed, recommendations for assessment need to be logical and logistically feasible. Multiple studies have attempted to delineate a set of demographic characteristics or medical diagnoses associated with victims of IPV. However, many abused women do not fit the demographic profiles developed and the lists of medical diagnoses are too long and diffuse to be useful. The evidence supports screening all women as opposed to screening only those with high-risk characteristics. There is no data available to judge the usefulness of assessing men or of screening for perpetrators. The concept of "universal screening" is often presented in an attempt to establish a screening protocol. The definitions of "universal screening" vary but often the term is used to indicate "screen every woman, every visit." A protocol based on this definition would fail to gain acceptance in the medical community. In primary care, patients are often seen every 4 to 6 weeks to adjust medications or follow up on chronic medical conditions. Frequent visits are also made for non-urgent conditions such as sore throats, ingrown toenails, and wart removal. To repeatedly ask patients about abuse with every visit would be senseless and a waste of time once the patient has been screened sufficiently. Medical providers are also asked to screen for a multitude of health risks, including cardiovascular disease, HIV disease, IPV, and alcohol and substance abuse. Providers cannot possibly screen for all these conditions on every single visit, and none of the disease prevention screenings can be viewed as preeminent. The data support screening every woman regardless of characteristics. Studies on pregnant women clearly support the need to assess for abuse more than once. The task, then, is to determine the optimal screening interval for all women throughout the lifecycle. Is it once a year, or once a year plus any injury visit, or every two years but more often in childbearing years? Further research is needed to answer these questions.

A related question: what is the optimal screening site? There is solid evidence that all women attending prenatal clinics need to be assessed for abuse in each trimester. Similarly, primary care offers an avenue for assessment of multiple health risks, including IPV. The evidence for screening all women or all persons entering the Emergency Department (ED) is less clear. Undeniably, a percentage of women who visit the ED are in abusive relationships. Some of these women present to the ED with injuries or other medical conditions that do not immediately raise the suspicion of IPV, occasionally even using the ED for primary care. However, no data exists to make a compelling case to screen all women who enter the ED regardless of presenting complaint. The argument could be made that in considering causes of morbidity and mortality in women, screening for smoking, risky sexual behavior, seat belt compliance, or breast health might be equally or more beneficial. The result would be an exhaustive, time consuming list of health risk screening that would overwhelm ED providers and potentially compromise the patient receiving needed acute care. This does not negate the importance of assessing for IPV in the ED but points to the need for further research into realistic assessment protocols given the morbidity and mortality risks to the lives of women and the nature of medical care in the ED.

INTERVENTION

Once a provider identifies a patient affected by IPV, a succinct and effective intervention must be readily available. Having a defined set of steps for intervention that can be realistically accomplished in a medical visit is crucial. To be realistic, the intervention must be short, starting with a basic "nuts and bolts" intervention that can be expanded as time allots. The intervention approach must be adaptable to a variety of practice settings, including private practice offices, emergency departments, and specialty clinics. Different practice sites will have different intervention priorities ranging from acute safety issues to treating long-term sequelae of previous abuse. The intervention components must be modifiable to meet the various clinical needs.

And again the intervention must be culturally appropriate. Tailoring an intervention toward leaving the abuser as the only option may be untenable to non-English speaking woman from an ethnic minority where leaving her abuser is synonymous with leaving her entire community. Interventions must take into account religious beliefs and the ability of some groups to effectively address IPV within their own cultural traditions. Qualitative research studies using focus groups and key informants are imperative for this process. While it is not feasible to do randomized controlled trials for every culturally distinct group, informed research can go a long way in providing important information to modify interventions to be culturally acceptable.

Several organizations provide clinical practice guidelines recommending intervention strategies using various combinations of the following four components: acknowledge the problem, assess safety, refer to appropriate resources, and provide good documentation (American College of Obstetricians and Gynecologists, 1995; American Medical Association, 1992; Family Violence Prevention Fund, found at www.fvpf.org). These components are logical and based on recommendations from expert panels and community service advocates. However, no data exists to define the best practice strategy or to verify the effectiveness of in-office intervention by a medical provider.

Several studies have examined interventions that are based in ambulatory settings or the emergency department (Krasnoff & Moscati, 2002; McFarlane, Parker, Soeken, & Bullock, 2000; McNutt, Carlson, Rose, & Robinson, 2002; Parker, McFarlane, Soeken, Conception, & Reel, 1999). The interventions often involve the use of on-site counselors or outreach case-managers. Many sites of practice may not have the personnel or financial resources to provide this level of intervention. Furthermore, many of the studies did not show a significant benefit over time to the intervention. However, McFarlane et al., Parker et al., and McNutt et al. all presented evidence that the simple act of assessing for abuse and providing access to IPV resource lists did decrease violence in the control groups.

The effectiveness of assessment and intervention in decreasing illness and injury due to IPV is truly the "black hole" from an evidence-based perspective. At this time, there exist general guidelines for appropriate intervention, well thought out by advocates, researchers, and medical providers, but with little or no data to support effectiveness. If physicians are going to be persuaded to invest time to assess and intervene with IPV, evidence of positive outcomes must be forthcoming.

What interventions work in the medical setting? What can medical providers do in an office visit that will have an impact on IPV? What support needs to be available on-site to increase the effectiveness of the intervention (social workers, community resource liaisons, case managers)? Determining what constitutes an intervention "working" is the first difficult task. What defines a positive outcome: an end to the violence, a reduction of injuries, improvement in mental well being, improvement in quality of life, the patient leaving the abusive situation, or the patient knowing the available options and resources? The goals of the medical provider may be different than the goals of the patient.

Through qualitative and quantitative research, the basic components of an effective intervention can be crafted.

Once the intervention is formulated and outcomes defined, longitudinal, randomized control trials of the intervention need to occur. Needless to say, this is an expensive undertaking. The studies require well thought out designs that ensure the safety of participants still in actively violent relationships. Data collection mechanisms must not require literacy, a telephone, or English as a first language. Qualitative and quantitative data collection will be required in order to understand not only the magnitude of the effect of the intervention but also the context of the outcomes. To ensure generalizability to multiple populations will require a large number of participants drawn form multiple study centers. And to be useful, the studies must be truly longitudinal. The outcomes for women need to be studied not just at 3 months or 6 months but also at 3 years and 6 years. This endeavor will require multiple agencies in multiple study sites combining resources and backed by sufficient funding to succeed.

EDUCATION

Although significant gaps in knowledge exist regarding IPV, medical providers still need to be educated regarding the medical consequences of IPV and offered the best known practices for assessment and intervention. Education cannot be put on hold pending the outcomes of multiple studies, some of which will require years to obtain useful data. Expert panels can draw upon clinical experience and currently published data to develop logical and reasonable guidelines.

One question is, "what is the best venue in which to educate physicians?" One obvious place to start is in medical school and residency. It is during training that physicians first learn interview skills and develop their sense of what constitutes important medical information. Knowledge of health risk assessment and preventative medicine is gained. Presenting the issues of IPV in a sensitive and informative manner is extremely important during this formative period.

A survey by Alpert, Tonkin, Seeherman, and Holtz (1998) found that 86% of deans reported inclusion of IPV teaching in their medical school curriculum; however, only 57% of students recalled learning about it. Residency training programs including training on IPV ranged from 40% in primary care (Staropoli, Moulton, & Cyr, 1997) to 80% in family practice (Rovi & Mouton, 1999). Varjavand, Cohen, and Novack

(2002) used standardized patients to assess the ability of residents to appropriately diagnose and manage a patient presenting with illness related to IPV. Over half (56%) correctly diagnosed IPV but 68% made at least one incorrect recommendation and 51% ordered unnecessary tests. Importantly, the 44% of residents who did not recognize IPV spent twice as much money on patient work-up. Clearly, many physicians will complete training with little or no training on IPV. Given the results of Varjavand's study, this lack of training will substantially increase medical care cost for victims of IPV as well as delay appropriate diagnosis and intervention.

Although many medical school and residency programs state that IPV is part of the curriculum, the nature of the training on IPV is not clear. Does training mean a one-hour didactic lecture during the first year of medical school with no ongoing reinforcement of the training? Studies have shown that without ongoing reinforcement, the improvement in screening and management brought about by an educational intervention will extinguish with time. In medical school and residency, it is essential that the importance of performing an abuse assessment be supported throughout the basic science as well as the clinical years. The enthusiasm and commitment to including an abuse assessment as an integral part of a medical history will wane if medical educators and attending physicians do not give it credence.

Often more challenging is to educate medical providers already in practice. Many were trained in a time when IPV was not considered part of the medical purview. Most struggle with the amount of new information they are required to absorb and apply. New treatments for HIV disease, heart failure, or diabetes often are viewed as more critical to learn than intervening with IPV. As many lecturers will attest, Continuing Medical Education conferences on IPV are well attended by nurses and social workers, but poorly attended by medical providers.

Several studies have attempted to test the effectiveness of a variety of educational approaches in changing medical providers' attitudes and/or behavior toward patients affected by IPV (Fanslow, Robinson, & Spinola, 1998; Harwell, Casten, Armstrong, Dempsey, Coons, & Davis, 1998; McCaw, Berman, Syme, & Hunkeler, 2001; Thompson et al., 2000). Each study trained staff using different combinations of didactics lectures, videos, role-playing, and presentations by survivors, community advocates, and prosecuting attorneys. Training involved 2 to 6 hours of staff time, either continuous or divided over several staff meetings. Possible systems changes included reminder stickers placed in charts, protocol development, direct feedback to providers regarding referral patterns, and newsletters with further educational information regarding IPV. Since each study chose different combinations of educational approaches and environmental prompts as well as different outcome measures, direct comparison is not possible. McCaw et al. found increased screening and improved HMO member satisfaction. McNutt et al. identified increased screening resulting in identification of severely abused women but also found an increase in patients accessing IPV patient education material. Harwell et al. found that although screening rates significantly increased, 75% of women were still not screened and the rates of documentation of IPV did not change. One of the more extensive interventions was performed by Thompson et al., who demonstrated a significant increase in provider self-efficacy but only a 14% increase in documentation of IPV screening and a 1.3 fold increase in case identification.

The outcomes for the above studies were modest. Furthermore, it is unclear which of the components most effectively changed providers' attitudes and screening/intervention behaviors. Thompson et al. (1998) presented data indicating providers highly rated the didactics with videos and role-playing. Survivors presentations were valued but less highly. Some of the interventions found significant drop-off of effect with time. Interventions must include not only an initial educational effort, but also ongoing reinforcement. Another difficulty is that many of the interventions were costly both in staff time required for training and in coordinating the environmental prompts such as reminder stickers in the chart, direct feedback, and newsletters. Many organizations do not have the staff and financial ability to carry out such an intensive intervention. Several of the interventions required on-site social workers or IPV liaisons that may not be readily available in some practice sites. An important step is to determine the most cost-effective, efficient, and efficacious intervention that improves providers' perceived self-efficacy, screening, and intervention practices, as well as case finding and documentation.

INSTITUTIONAL SUPPORT

For medical providers to succeed in diagnosing and intervening with IPV, institutional support is crucial. A cultural norm of responding to IPV is more likely to exist if clinic and hospital administrators endorse IPV as an important medical issue. Beyond endorsing is pro-actively assisting medical providers to increase the likelihood of successful interventions. Many IPV trainers have encountered administrators who verbally and enthusiastically acknowledge the importance of IPV training but fail to provide concrete help with setting aside in-service time or funding needed system changes to ensure success.

In order to enlist the support of administrators, providing evidence of the cost of undiagnosed IPV is often helpful. Kernic, Wol, and Holt (2000) analyzed hospitalization rates of abused women in the year prior to filing a protection order compared with non-abused women. The study showed an increase relative risk of hospitalization for abused women ranging from 1.2 in older women to 2.1 in women age 18-24. Specific diagnoses, psychiatric diagnosis (RR = 3.6), assault (RR = 4.9) and suicide attempts (RR = 3.7) revealed a marked increase risk. Ulrich, Cain, Sugg, Rivara, Rubanowice, and Thompson (2003) found that abused women had 7.2 more total visits per year resulting in $1,722 more money spent on health care services compared to non-abused women. Varjavand et al. (2002) found that residents who failed to correctly diagnose IPV spent nearly twice as much on work-up compared to residents who made the diagnosis. There is ample documentation that women in abuse situations have higher medical utilization. Less clear is the effect of diagnosis on the pattern of utilization. It is conceivable that cost and utilization may initially increase post-diagnosis as more services are needed during the intervention phase. Ultimately, the cost and utilization may decrease if the IPV ceases but there is no data to determine if this is the case.

Another factor influencing administrators is regulatory over-site by accreditation organizations such as Joint Commission on Accreditation of Healthcare Organizations. (JCAHO). JCAHO requires protocols to be developed to identify victims of abuse. Preparation for JCAHO or other over-site surveys presents an opportunity to advocate for resources that improve care for patients affected by violence. Swenson-Britt, Thornton, and Brackley (2001) describes the step by step use of the continuous improvement process (CIP) model to bring about multiple system changes resulting in improved medical documentation and a more coordinated system of response for abused patients, Dienemann and colleagues (2002) designed an IPV critical pathway for use in geographically diverse hospitals. The critical pathway was developed by an interdisciplinary panel of experts to ensure scientific accuracy and logistic feasibility and included input from battered women. This pathway encompasses physical, mental, and social assessment and treatment to decrease treatment variability and improve overall quality. Once a system-wide protocol exists, gaps in services or areas of needed improvement can be more readily identified and continuously improved upon. This process, although more time consuming, leads to a more seamless response than piecemeal improvements that often occur in isolation.

PROFESSIONAL ORGANIZATION SUPPORT

In the early 1990s, the American Medical Association (AMA; 1992) disseminated guidelines for identification and intervention of domestic violence. This document provided an excellent starting place for standardization of care for patients affected by IPV. In the interim, many other organizations (American Medical Association, American Academy of Family Physicians, American Academy of Pediatrics, American College of Emergency Physicians, American College of Obstetricians and Gynecologists) have also developed practice guidelines and championed the issue of IPV, recognizing the profound effect violence has on the lives of patients (Rhodes & Levinson, 2003). Many of these organizations have invested time and money to develop educational and referral information to assist their members. A few have developed web sites that provide immediate access to crucial information for busy practitioners (www.acep.org, www.acog.org). The Family Violence Prevention Fund is a national organization dedicated to preventing family violence through education and advocacy. The FVPF offers a wealth of information, resources, and support for medical providers readily accessible on their web site (www.fvpf.org).

The support of professional organizations is key for a variety of reasons. The obvious is the ability to reach a large number of medical providers with educational materials. Equally important, professional organizations are well placed to influence governmental decisions regarding funding for violence prevention initiative, prioritizing federal research dollars, and strengthening laws that aid abuse victims. But perhaps most importantly, through policy statements and development of standards, professional organizations gradually change the medical culture to recognize the importance of responding to IPV.

RESEARCH SUPPORT

Recently, the U.S. Preventive Services Task Force (USPSTF) reviewed the literature on intimate partner violence and gave a grade I recommendation, finding insufficient evidence for or against routine screening of women for intimate partner violence (U.S. Preventive Services Task Force, 2004). Furthermore, the task force found no evidence that screening for IPV decreased disability or premature death and limited evidence that intervention reduced harm to women. The USPSTF has a rigorous protocol for evaluating the quality of randomized controlled trials and cohort and case-control studies, with emphasis on well-designed controlled trials in representative populations (Nelson, Nygren, McInerney, & Klein, 2004.) The Canadian Task Force on Preventive Health Care made similar recommendations after their own rigorous review of the literature (MacMillan & Wathen, 2001; Wathen & MacMillan, 2003).

However, these task force recommendations rely heavily on controlled trials of large populations and do not take into account the wealth of knowledge and experiences of experts in the field. As Dr. Lachs (2004) so eloquently states in his editorial, " . . . perhaps the type of evidence we demand for this kind of healing should be different from what we demand for the efficacy of anticoagulation in atrial fibrillation" (p. 400). Obviously, providers cannot wait 10 years to have all the questions answered through longitudinal research. Patients affected by violence present to exam rooms in every clinical setting every minute of every day. Medical providers must have a starting place for responding while awaiting further support from clinical studies.

The groundwork laid by the development of guidelines and critical pathways needs to be expanded into a national expert panel consensus statement. The strength of consensus statements over guidelines is that consensus statements present the outcomes benefited and the strength of the evidence that supports each recommendation. Consensus statements exist for asthma, hypertension, HIV treatment, diabetes, and many other medical conditions. Many, like the Seventh Report of the Joint National Committee on Detection, Evaluation, and Treatment of High Blood Pressure (JNC 7), provide updated recommendations every 3 to 5 years as the research advances (Chobanian et al., 2003). Given the vast number of studies to be reviewed, some with conflicting results, medical providers often are not in a position to rigorously review all the data for a given medical problem. Medical providers rely on these consensus statements to present in a concise manner the state of knowledge for a particular disease process and delineate acceptable medical practices. Equally important is the frequent revision of the consensus statement to reflect new knowledge gained in ongoing research.

Of interest in examining existing consensus documents for other diseases are how often recommendations are not supported by randomized control trials, cohort, or case studies. The recommendations are put forth based on clinical experience and best extrapolation from existing data by the consensus panel. In the field of IPV, medical providers, researchers, and advocates can bring to bear their vast experience with abuse victims in formulating recommendations and be on par with other well-respected consensus panels.

Multiple benefits ensue from a consensus statement. Training of medical providers is easier with documentation of evidenced-based recommendations. The consensus statements can be disseminated via the Web, thereby being more accessible to healthcare providers. Gaps in research are more readily identified when existing studies have been reviewed and evaluated by an expert panel. Final, patients will benefit from a standard of care that reflects the best medical knowledge.

CONCLUSION

Many lives are damaged or destroyed each day by IPV. Physicians and mid-level practitioners are in key positions to help patients affected by violence. However, medical providers need appropriate tools (a validated assessment instrument and effective intervention protocol) and multiple layers of support (institutional, professional, and personal) to succeed. Domestic violence advocates, survivors, medical providers, and researchers all have important roles in educating and galvanizing the medical profession in its response to IPV.

REFERENCES

Abbott, J., Johnson, R., Koziol-McLain, J., & Lowenstein, S. R. (1995). Domestic violence against women. Incidence and prevalence in an emergency department population. *Journal of the American Medical Association, 273*, 1763-1767.

Alpert, E. J., Tonkin, A. E., Seeherman, A. M., & Holtz, H. A. (1998). Family violence curricula in U.S. medical schools. *American Journal Preventative Medicine, 12*, 273-282.

American College of Obstetricians and Gynecologists. (1995). ACOG issues technical bulletin on domestic violence. *American Family Physician, 52*, 2387-2388, 2391.

American Medical Association. (1992). *Diagnostic and treatment guidelines on domestic violence.* Chicago, IL: Author.

Beck, S. R., Freitag, S. K., & Singer, N. (1996). Ocular injuries in battered women. *Ophthalmology, 103*, 148-151.

Campbell J. C., & Lewandowski, L. A. (1997). Mental and physical health effects of intimate partner violence on women and children. *Psychiatric Clinics of North America, 20*(2), 353-374.

Campbell, J., Jones, A., Dienemann, J., Kub, J., Schollenberger, J., O'Campo, P. et al. (2002). Intimate partner violence and physical health consequences. *Archives of Internal Medicine, 162*, 1157-1163.

Cascardi, M., Langhinrichsen, J., & Vivian, D. (1992). Marital aggression: Impact, injury, and health correlates for husbands and wives. *Archives of Internal Medicine, 152*, 1178-1184.

Cascardi, M., Mueser, K. T., DeGiralomo, J., & Murrin, M. (1996). Physical aggression against psychiatric inpatients by family members and partners. *Psychiatric Services, 47*(5), 531-533.

Chobanian, A., Bakris, G., Black, H., Cushman, W., Green, L., Izzo, J. et al. (2003). The seventh report of the Joint National Committee on prevention, detection, evaluation, and treatment of high blood pressure. *Journal of the American Medical Association, 289*(19), 2560-2572.

Danielson, K., Moffitt, T., Caspi, A., & Silva, P. (1998). Comorbidity between abuse of an adult and DSM-III-R mental disorders: Evidence from an epidemiological study. *American Journal of Psychiatry, 155*, 131-133.

Dienemann, J., Campbell, J., Wiederhorn, N., Laughon, K., & Jordan, E. (2002). A critical pathway for intimate partner violence across the continuum of care. *Journal of Obstetric, Gynecologic, and Neonatal Nursing, 32*, 594-603.

Domino, J. V., & Haber, J. D. (1987). Prior physical and sexual abuse in women with chronic headaches: Clinical correlates. *Headache, 27*(6), 310-314.

Drossman, D. A., Leserman, J., Nachman, G., Li, Z. M., Gluck, H., & Toomey, T. C. (1990). Sexual and physical abuse in women with functional or organic gastrointestinal disorders. *Annals of Internal Medicine, 113*, 828-833.

Ernst, A., Weiss, S., Cham, E., & Marquez, M. (2002). Comparison of three instruments for assessing ongoing intimate partner violence. *Medical Science Monitor: International Medical Journal of Experimental and Clinical Research, 8*(3), 197-201.

Fairchild, D., Fairchild, M. W., & Stoner, S. (1998). Prevalence of adult domestic violence among women seeking routine care in a Native American health care facility. *American Journal of Public Health, 88*, 1515-1517.

Family Violence Prevention Fund, www.fvpf.org.

Fanslow, J., Robinson, E., & Spinola, C. (1998). Outcome evaluation of an emergency department protocol of care on partner abuse. *Australian and New Zealand Journal of Public Health, 22*(5), 598-603.

Feldhaus, K. M., Koziol-McLain, J., Amsbury, H., Norton, I., Lowenstein, S., & Abbott, J. (1997). Accuracy of 3 brief screening questions for detecting intimate partner violence in the emergency department. *Journal of the American Medical Association, 277*(17), 1357-1361.

Gazmararian, J., Lazorick, S., Spitz, A., Ballard, T., Saltzman, L., & Marks, J. (1996). Prevalence of violence against pregnant women. *Journal of the American Medical Association, 275*, 1915-1920.

Gin, N. E., Ruker, L., Frayne, S., Cygan, R., & Hubbell, F. A. (1991). Prevalence of domestic violence among patients in three ambulatory care internal medicine clinics. *Journal of General Internal Medicine, 6*, 317-322.

Haber, J. D., & Roos, C. (1985). Effects of spouse abuse in the development and maintenance of chronic pain in women. *Advances in Pain Research, 9,* 889-895.

Hamberger, L. K., Saunders, D. G., & Hovey, M. (1992). Prevalence of domestic violence in community practice and rate of physician inquiry. *Family Medicine, 24,* 283-287.

Harwell, T. S., Casten, R. J., Armstrong, K. A., Dempsey, S., Coons, H. L., & Davis, M. D. (1998). Results of a domestic violence training program offered to the staff of urban community health centers. *American Journal of Preventative Medicine, 15*(3), 235-242.

Jacobson, A., & Richardson, B. (1987). Assault experiences of 100 psychiatric inpatients: Evidence of the need for routine inquiry. *American Journal of Psychiatry, 144,* 908-913.

Johnson, M., & Elliott, B. (1997). Domestic violence among family practice patients in midsized and rural communities. *Journal of Family Practice, 44,* 391-400.

Kernic, M., Wol, M., & Holt, V. (2000). Rates and relative risk of hospital admission among women in violent intimate partner relationships. *American Journal of Public Health, 90,* 1416-1420.

Krasnoff, M., & Moscati, R. (2002). Domestic violence screening and referral can be effective. *Annals of Emergency Medicine, 40,* 485-492.

Lachs, M. S. (2004). Screening for family violence: What's an evidence-based doctor to do? *Annals of Internal Medicine, 140*(5), 399-400.

Le, B., Dierks, E., Ueeck, B., Homer, L., & Potter, B. (2001). Maxillofacial injuries associated with domestic violence. *Journal of Oral Maxillofacial Surgery, 59,* 1277-1283.

MacMillan, H. L., & Wathen C. N., with the Canadian Task Force on Preventive Health Care. (2001). Prevention and treatment of violence against women. In *Systematic review & recommendations.* London, Ontario: Canadian Task Force. CTFPHC Technical Report No. 01-4.

McCauley, J., Kern, D., Kolodner, K., Dill, L., Schroeder, A., DeChant, H. et al. (1995). The "battering syndrome": Prevalence and clinical characteristics of domestic violence in primary care internal medicine practices. *Annals Internal Medicine, 123,* 737-746.

McCaw, B., Berman, W., Syme, L., & Hunkeler, E. (2001). Beyond screening for domestic violence: A systems model approach in a managed care setting. *American Journal of Preventative Medicine, 21*(3), 170-176.

McFarlane, J., Parker, B., Soeken, K., & Bullock, L. (1992). Assessing for abuse during pregnancy. *Journal of the American Medical Association, 267*(23), 3176-3178.

McFarlane, J., Soeken, K., & Wiist, W. (2000). An evaluation of interventions to decrease intimate partner violence to pregnant women. *Public Health Nursing, 17*(6), 443-451.

McNutt, L. A., Carlson, B. E., Rose, I. M., & Robinson, D. A. (2002). Partner violence intervention in the busy primary care environment. *American Journal of Preventative Medicine, 22*(2), 82-91.

Nelson, H., Nygren, P., McInerney, Y., & Klein, J. (2004). Screening women and elderly adults for family and intimate partner violence: A review of the evidence for the U.S. Preventive Services Task Force. *Annals of Internal Medicine, 140,* 387-396.

Parker, B., McFarlane, J., Soeken, K., Conception, S., & Reel, S. (1999). Testing an intervention to prevent further abuse to pregnant women. *Research in Nursing and Health, 22*, 59-66.

Perciaccante, V., Ochs, H., & Dodson, T. (1999). Head, neck and facial injuries as markers of domestic violence in women. *Journal of Oral Maxillofacial Surgery, 57*, 760-762.

Rath, G. D., Jarrett, L. G., & Leonardson, G. (1989). Rates of domestic violence against adult women by men partners. *Journal of the American Board of Family Practice, 2*, 227-233.

Rhodes, K., & Levinson, W. (2003) Interventions for intimate partner violence against women. Clinical applications. *Journal of the American Medical Association, 289*(5), 601-605.

Roberts, G., O'Toole, B., Raphael, B., Lawrence, J., & Ashby, R. (1996). Prevalence study of domestic violence victims in an emergency department. *Annals of Emergency Medicine, 27*(6), 747-753.

Rovi, M., & Mouton, C. P. (1999). Domestic violence education in family practice residencies. *Family Medicine, 31*, 398-403.

Sherin, K., Sinacore, J., Li, X. Q., Zitter, R., & Shakil, A. (1998). HITS: A short domestic violence screening tool for use in a family practice setting. *Family Medicine 30*(7), 508-512.

Staropoli, C. A., Moulton, A. W., & Cyr, M. G. (1997). Primary care internal medicine training and women's health. *Journal of General Internal Medicine, 12*, 129-131.

Swenson-Britt, E., Thornton, J., & Brackley, M. (2001). A continuous improvement process of health providers of victims of domestic violence. *The Joint Commission Journal on Quality Improvement, 27*(10), 540-554.

Thompson, R. S., Meyer, B. A., Smith-DiJulio, K., Caplow, M. P., Maiuro, R. D., Thompson, D.C. et al. (1998). A training program to improve domestic violence identification and management in primary care: Preliminary results. *Violence Victims, 13*(4), 395-410.

Thompson, R. S., Rivara, F. P., Thompson, D. C., Barlow, W. E., Sugg, N. K., Maiuro, R. D. et al. (2000). Identification and management of domestic violence: A randomized trial. *American Journal of Preventative Medicine, 19*(4), 253-263.

Ulrich, Y., Cain, K., Sugg, N., Rivara, F., Rubanowice, D., & Thompson, R. (2003). Medical care utilization patterns in women with diagnosed domestic violence. *American Journal of Preventative Medicine, 24*(1), 9-15.

U.S. Preventive Services Task Force. (2004). Screening for family and intimate partner violence: Recommendation statement. *Annals of Internal Medicine, 140*, 382-386.

Varjavand, N., Cohen, D., & Novack, D. (2002). An assessment of residents' abilities to detect and manage domestic violence. *Journal of General Internal Medicine, 17*, 465-468.

Wathen, C. N., & MacMillan, H. (2003). Interventions for violence against women. Scientific review. *Journal of the American Medical Association, 289*(5), 589-600.

Young, M. E., Nosek, M. A., Howland, C., Chanpong, G., & Rintala, D. (1997). Prevalence of abuse of women with physical disabilities. *Archives of Physical Medicine Rehabilitation, 8*, S34-S38.

Zachariades, N., Koumoura, F., & Konsolaki-Agouridaki, E. (1990). Facial trauma in women resulting from violence by men. *Journal of Oral Maxillofacial Surgery, 48*, 1250-1253.

doi:10.1300/J146v13n03_05

CHANGING THE WAY YOUNG PEOPLE HANDLE ANGER AND INTERACT WITH THEIR INTIMATE PARTNERS

Can We Prevent the Hitting? Recommendations for Preventing Intimate Partner Violence Between Young Adults

K. Daniel O'Leary
Erica M. Woodin
Patti A. T. Fritz

SUMMARY. All empirically-evaluated partner violence prevention programs were reviewed. Most changed knowledge and attitudes regarding dating and sexual aggression, but few demonstrated behavioral change. Peer violence and substance use programs directed toward at-risk individuals demonstrate much larger effects than those directed at all individuals. Research is needed to (a) identify risk-factors for vio-

Address correspondence to K. Daniel O'Leary, PhD, Psychology Department, Stony Brook University, Stony Brook, NY 11794 (E-mail: K.D.OLeary@sunysb.edu).

This work was supported in part by a Department of Defense Contract, NIMH Grant #57985 awarded to K. Daniel O'Leary, and a Stony Brook University Graduate Council Fellowship awarded to the second author.

[Haworth co-indexing entry note]: "Can We Prevent the Hitting? Recommendations for Preventing Intimate Partner Violence Between Young Adults." O'Leary, K. Daniel, Erica M. Woodin, and Patti A. T. Fritz. Co-published simultaneously in *Journal of Aggression, Maltreatment & Trauma* (The Haworth Maltreatment & Trauma Press, an imprint of The Haworth Press, Inc.) Vol. 13, No. 3/4, 2006, pp. 121-178; and: *Prevention of Intimate Partner Violence* (ed: Sandra M. Stith) The Haworth Maltreatment & Trauma Press, an imprint of The Haworth Press, Inc., 2006, pp. 121-178. Single or multiple copies of this article are available for a fee from The Haworth Document Delivery Service [1-800-HAWORTH, 9:00 a.m. - 5:00 p.m. (EST). E-mail address: docdelivery@haworthpress.com].

lence persistence, (b) examine the cost-benefit of universal and targeted programs, and (c) explore the ability of programs, such as parenting, stress management, and substance abuse programs, to reduce partner aggression. We recommend that institutions implement hierarchical systems of prevention, with brief interventions for all; more extensive program for moderate levels of aggression; and intensive psychosocial and legal interventions for serious offenders. doi:10.1300/J146v13n03_06 *[Article copies available for a fee from The Haworth Document Delivery Service: 1-800-HAWORTH. E-mail address: <docdelivery@haworthpress.com> Website: <http://www.HaworthPress.com> © 2006 by The Haworth Press, Inc. All rights reserved.]*

KEYWORDS. Prevention, violence, aggression, partner, intervention, treatment

This article provides a review of prevention programs to reduce physical aggression against partners, and offers recommendations for future prevention initiatives. We begin by presenting an overview of the prevalence of and risk factors for physical aggression against partners, with a special focus on aggression in young adults. We then present a rationale for the need for prevention of physical aggression against partners and a summary of published programs designed to reduce such aggression.

Because there are relatively few published prevention studies in this area, we also review prevention programs designed to reduce sexual aggression, substance abuse, and acting-out behavior in young adults–antisocial behaviors that often co-occur with partner aggression. These prevention areas are reviewed not only because they are generally correlated with physical aggression against partners, but also because these programs are numerous, well developed, and are often summarized in meta-analytic outcome reviews. Moreover, the strategies from these prevention areas that are most effective in reducing various types of acting out behaviors appear relevant to the problem of partner aggression. We therefore conclude the article by offering recommendations for future partner aggression prevention initiatives by drawing both from the dating and sexual aggression prevention literatures and from research conducted in these related prevention areas. More specifically, we present a tiered approach to the prevention of partner aggression.

PREVALENCE AND CORRELATES
OF PARTNER AGGRESSION

Physical aggression against partners in the United States occurs at rates higher than most laypersons and professionals expect. Acts of physical aggression by men against their intimate partners, such as pushing, slapping, shoving, and hitting, are reported by 12% of women in the United States each year (Straus & Gelles, 1990). Perhaps not surprisingly, as relationships begin to become problematic in young couples, the frequency of arguing, and, in turn, physical aggression increases (O'Leary, Barling, Arias, Rosenbaum, Malone, & Tyree, 1989). Approximately 50-60% of couples in troubled marriages report the presence of physical aggression (Holtzworth-Munroe, Waltz, Jacobson, Monaco, Fehrenbach, & Gottman, 1992; O'Leary, Vivian, & Malone, 1992).

One of the best predictors of all types of aggression is age (Wilson & Hernstein, 1985). More specifically, aggression of almost all varieties is more common in young adults than in middle age and older people. For example, assault and rape occur most frequently in men between their late teens and late twenties (Wilson & Herrnstein, 1985). Similarly, physical aggression against intimate partners occurs most frequently in the late teens and twenties (O'Leary, 1999). Examination of age trends across the decades from early adolescence to the eighties reveals an inverted U shaped curve with physical aggression in intimate relationships occurring at low rates in the early teens, rising rapidly into the mid-twenties, and declining thereafter. At the highest point, approximately 35%-40% of women report that their partners engaged in some act of physical aggression against them in the past year. The majority of such aggression is not severe aggression. Most commonly, it is slapping, pushing, shoving, and hitting. The more severe forms of partner aggression, such as beating up or using a knife or gun against a partner, occur in less than 1% of a community samples of young married couples, but such aggression becomes more common as relationships deteriorate (e.g., O'Leary et al., 1989).

These above mentioned age trends in physical aggression might lead some to believe that aggressive individuals cease engaging in acts of physical aggression as they get older. Indeed, based on cross sectional data, many men and women appear to cease being aggressive as they age (Feld & Straus, 1989). Our follow-up of women a decade after marriage showed that the majority of couples from a community sample ceased engaging in physical aggression. At pre-marriage, 27% of the women reported that their partners engaged in physical aggression against them, but a decade later only 10% of the wives reported that their partners continued to engage in such aggression (Fritz & O'Leary, 2004). However, when we assessed for the occurrence of physical aggression across repeated time periods in this same sample of young newlyweds, about half of the men continued to engage in acts of aggression at all four assessment periods across the first 30 months of marriage (Lorber & O'Leary, 2004). Taken together, these findings suggest that while couples who are aggressive premaritally tend to remain consistently aggressive in the early years of marriage, many couples discontinue their use of physical aggression by the end of the first decade of marriage.

A number of other risk factors for partner aggression also have been identified, including a history of family disruption and violence (Dutton, 1988; Widom, 1989), witnessing or directly experiencing violence as a child (e.g., Wekerle & Wolfe, 1999), acceptance of male violence, gender inequality, and patriarchal social institutions (Dobash & Dobash, 1979; Yllo, 1993), and having traditional sex role attitudes (Finn, 1986). Further risk-factors include negative affect (e.g., insults, disagreeableness), coercive negotiation styles, confrontational coping (Bird, Stith, & Schladale, 1991; Laner, 1989), limited social support coping (Bird et al., 1991), and high levels of jealousy, dominance tactics, anger, and a reported need for control (Boyle & Vivian, 1996; Burcky, Reuterman, & Kopsky, 1988; Cate, Henton, Koval, Christopher, & Lloyd, 1982; Dutton, 1988; Follingstad, Wright, Lloyd, & Sebastian, 1991; Matthews, 1984).

In addition, a strong and consistent association has been shown between alcohol abuse and interpartner violence (Bogal-Allbritten & Allbritten, 1985; Carlson, 1987; Laner, 1983; Makepeace, 1981; O'Keeffe, Brockopp, & Chew, 1986; Roscoe & Callahan, 1985). Self-reported problems with alcohol increased the risk of severe partner aggression in Army personnel by 121% (Pan, Neidig, & O'Leary, 1994). Although alcohol use does not always occur with partner violence, it has been associated with serious injury (Martin & Bachman, 1997). Furthermore, given that alcohol use is so prevalent among adolescents and young adults, this association is of great concern. In sum, a number of behavioral and personality variables have been found to be associated with partner violence.

Given such risk factors, it is apparent that partner violence prevention programs must target a wide variety of empirically identified behaviors and skill deficits. Programs should, for instance, address sex roles and issues of power and control with regard to intimate relationships, and include conflict management and communication skills training. Prevention programs should also address substance use/abuse issues, and the link between partner violence and substance use. We now turn to various prevention strategies, their rationales, and how risk factors can be used to select the particular prevention strategy.

EFFORTS TO PREVENT PARTNER AGGRESSION

Prevention efforts can be universal or targeted at populations at risk. Universal prevention programs are broad-based and directed at all individuals in a population such as a whole high school, all men and women in their first year at a college or university, or all recruits at a military base. Universal programs are administered independent of risk status, and thus avoid possible labeling or stigmatization that could be associated with selecting a segment of a population (Greenberg, Domitrovich, & Bumbarger, 2001). Targeted prevention programs are directed at individuals that appear to be at higher risk than the average person, such as those experiencing marital discord or problematic alcohol use. Such populations might include individuals arrested for disorderly conduct or individuals who have impulse control problems manifested in a variety of ways (e.g., speeding, driving while intoxicated, aggressive personality style, high levels of psychological abuse and controlling behavior, or a history of fighting outside the home).

Prevention need not occur only at one level. Indeed, from a broad social perspective, unless there is evidence that a prevention effort produces an iatrogenic effect, it seems quite appropriate to address any problem from various vantage points. For example, we later review universal prevention efforts to reduce smoking, and, as you will see, some of those efforts have not demonstrated significant effects compared to no-treatment control groups. However, the programs designed to prevent or reduce smoking did not occur in a vacuum. They occurred at a time of significant social change, when legal efforts caused smoking to be less likely in many public places, taxes for tobacco products increased markedly, and there were frequent public disclosures of individuals who lost loved ones to lung cancer and other smoking-related diseases. In short, smoking prevention programs have been taking place in a larger social context in which attempts to prevent or stop smoking have occurred from many different vantage points.

Prevention of partner aggression and attempts to curb ongoing partner abuse also have the potential to occur on various levels. Examples of such varied interventions might include: public service announcements with phone numbers of hotlines and service agencies, elementary and secondary school-based prevention efforts for all students in the schools, programs for couples with relationship problems, programs for men and/or women who abuse alcohol or other substances, or programs for fathers and mothers with serious discipline problems (since they are at high risk for both child and partner abuse; O'Leary & Woodin, 2005).

Prevention Strategies to Motivate Behaviors Conducive to Reducing Partner Abuse

We believe that individuals will seek help for problems that are beginning to cause them significant concern, and generally not before then. For example, individuals generally do not seek help from physicians for means of lowering their blood pressure or weight until they experience problems such as dizziness or lack of energy. Similarly, individuals do not generally seek out preventative services for partner abuse. In fact, even when such services were offered free of charge, few couples responded to our advertisements for a program to prevent marital discord and partner aggression (Holtzworth-Munroe et al., 1995). Individuals generally seek out services when the problems they are facing begin to cause them significant distress. One means of dealing with this dilemma is to provide services for individuals at risk for partner aggression when they see a professional such as a physician for an annual physical, especially if the physician routinely asks if there is any physical aggression in a relationship (as is the case for many military physicians). Similarly, gynecologists might assess for partner abuse and make appropriate referrals since they see women at peak ages for partner abuse. Finally, partner abuse prevention services may also be provided to couples who have marital problems. In short, provision of services for individuals at risk for partner aggression could be offered in the context of other service provisions.

Given the relatively high prevalence of partner violence, especially among young adults in their late teens and twenties, and the lack of attention to and published evaluations of controlled outcome partner violence prevention programs, a great need for prevention efforts in this area exists. Thus, the remainder of this article will be organized around two major areas: (a) the review of empirically evaluated prevention programs for dating and sexual violence, and (b) the review of programs designed to reduce delinquent behavior and substance abuse. The latter review is presented because there are only nine published controlled outcome studies in the field of partner abuse prevention. Further, since prevention research has been so voluminous in the substance abuse area, it seemed important to ascertain what has been learned in that arena, particularly since alcohol and drug abuse have highly significant links to partner aggression and other forms of antisocial behavior (e.g., Schumacher, Feldbau-Kohn, Slep, & Heyman, 2001).

DATING AND SEXUAL VIOLENCE PREVENTION PROGRAMS

Overview of Violence Prevention Programs

Despite the prevalence of dating violence, relatively few empirical studies have evaluated universal or targeted prevention programs for dating violence among unmarried individuals. Of the few studies that have been published, nearly all are of school-based programs involving junior high and high school students (Avery-Leaf, Cascardi, O'Leary, & Cano, 1997; Foshee et al., 2000; Jaffe, Sudermann, Reitzel, & Killip, 1992; Jones, 1991; Krajewski, Rybarik, Dosch, & Gilmore, 1996; Lavoie, Vézina, Piché, & Boivin, 1995; Macgowan, 1997; Weisz & Black, 2001; Wolfe et al., 2003).

In fact, only one controlled outcome study involving the recruit of unmarried young adults has been published. Markman, Renick, Floyd, Stanley, and Clements (1993) evaluated the Prevention and Relationship Enhancement Program (PREP), a 5-session program used to teach couples effective communication and conflict management skills. Community couples planning marriage for the first time were recruited. Long-term follow-up results indicated that up to four years following the end of the program, "couples showed greater use of communication skills, greater positive affect, more problem solving skill, more support and validation, less withdrawal, less denial, less dominance, less conflict, and less overall negative communication than did control couples at the same time" (p. 75). PREP also reduced the tendency to resort to physical violence and to dissolve relationships among participants in the intervention group. However, by the five-year follow-up, many of the effects had diminished. In fact, the only variable that intervention couples differed significantly from control couples on at the five-year follow-up was communication skills usage by men.

Furthermore, the results on the PREP program may not generalize to a non-research environment since the participants were initially recruited and paid as participants in a study of marriage. Then, once the couples were in the study, they were offered the possibility of participating in a program for enhancing the marriage. In short, while results from PREP appear promising despite several limitations, essentially no other empirical data exist on the effectiveness of physical dating violence prevention programs with unmarried adults. Given the dearth of research on young adult dating or married partners, the literature surrounding the prevention of physical dating violence among adolescents will be reviewed. In addition, the sexual assault prevention literature will also be reviewed. It should be noted, however, that unlike the physical dating aggression programs, the majority of sexual assault prevention programs have been implemented with unmarried young adults (i.e., college students).

Adolescent Dating Violence and Young Adult Sexual Assault Prevention Programs

Numerous adolescent dating and sexual violence programs exist across the United States and Canada. In fact, organizations such as the Office of Community Services Administration for Children and Families (1997) have published lists of dating violence programs for schools. However, relatively few programs have been empirically evaluated, and only a handful of evaluations have been published. Of the dating violence programs that have been evaluated and published, eight are universal dating prevention programs and one program is designed for adolescents with a childhood history of maltreatment (a targeted prevention program). Of the sexual assault prevention programs, 35 programs are universal in nature and two are targeted at high-risk males (Schewe & O'Donohue, 1993, 1996) and three are targeted at women with a history of sexual victimization (Breitenbecher & Gidycz, 1998; Himelein, 1999; Marx, Calhoun, Wilson, & Meyerson, 2001).

In reviewing these evaluations, similarities in the programs emerge. First, most of the adolescent dating violence and young adult sexual assault prevention programs possess both a didactic and process-oriented, skills-based approach (e.g., Avery-Leaf et al., 1997; Breitenbecher & Scarce, 1999; Foubert & McEwen, 1998; Gidycz, Lynn et al., 2001; Himelein, 1999; Krajewski et al., 1996; Macgowan, 1997; Marx et al., 2001; Rosenthal, Heesacker, & Neimeyer, 1995; Weisz & Black, 2001; Wolfe et al., 1996). Several of the sexual assault prevention programs also utilize videotaped (Anderson, Stoelb, Duggan, Hieger, Kling, & Payne, 1998; Breitenbecher & Gidycz, 1998; Fonow, Richardson, & Wemmerus, 1992; Foubert, 2000; Foubert & Marriott, 1997; Foubert & McEwen, 1998; Gidycz, Lynn et al., 2001; Hanson & Gidycz, 1993; Harrison, Downes, & Williams, 1991; Heppner, Humphrey, Hillenbrand-Gunn, & DeBord, 1995; Heppner, Good et al., 1995; Heppner, Neville, Smith, Kivlighan, & Gershuny, 1999; Lenihan, Rawlins, Eberly, Buckley, & Masters, 1992; Linz, Fuson, & Donnerstein, 1990; Lonsway et al., 1998; Lonsway & Kothari, 2000; Marx et al., 2001; Nelson & Torgler, 1990; Patton & Mannison, 1993; Schewe & O'Donohue, 1993, 1996) or theatrical (Black, Weisz, Coats, & Patterson, 2000; Frazier, Valtinson, & Candell, 1994; Heppner, Humphrey et al., 1995; Heppner et al., 1999; Lanier, Elliott, Martin, & Kapadia, 1998) presentations as the media of implementation for these approaches.

Second, the basic objectives of the dating violence and sexual assault prevention programs tend to overlap. For instance, a key focus of essentially all of the prevention programs is to promote equity in dating relationships and to challenge gender stereotypes and sexist attitudes that perpetuate physical and sexual violence. In addition, nearly all of the programs aim to increase participants' knowledge about the importance of the problem of dating and sexual violence in relationships, the various kinds and levels of abuse and intimidation, the early warning signs of abusive patterns in relationships, and the availability of community resources for both victims and perpetrators of dating and sexual violence (e.g., Avery-Leaf et al., 1997; Breitenbecher & Gidycz, 1998; Breitenbecher & Scarce, 1999; Gidycz, Lynn et al., 2001; Hanson & Gidycz, 1993; Jaffe et al., 1992; Jones, 1991; Lonsway & Kothari, 2000; Pinzone-Glover, Gidycz, & Jacobs, 1998). Three of the dating violence programs (Avery-Leaf et al., 1997; Foshee et al., 1996; Wolfe et al., 2003) and 11 of the sexual assault programs (Breitenbecher & Gidycz, 1998; Breitenbecher & Scarce, 1999, 2001; Foubert, 2000; Gidycz, Layman et al., 2001; Gidycz, Lynn et al., 2001; Gray, Lesser, Quinn, & Bounds, 1990; Hanson & Gidycz, 1993; Linz et al., 1990; Marx et al., 2001; Schewe & O'Donohue, 1993) also sought to decrease perpetration and/or victimization of partner violence. Similarly, several of the programs also include identifying and improving constructive communication and conflict management skills (Avery-Leaf et al., 1997; Breitenbecher & Gidycz, 1998; Breitenbecher & Scarce, 2001; Foshee et al., 1996; Gidycz, Lynn et al., 2001; Hanson & Gidycz, 1993; Jones, 1991; Krajewski et al., 1996; Macgowan, 1997; Marx et al., 2001; Wolfe et al., 1996), and strengthening communication and interaction between families, students, schools, and the surrounding community as objectives (Foshee et al., 1996; Jaffe et al., 1992). In short, many of the adolescent dating violence and young adult sexual assault prevention programs appear very similar. The similarities among the physical and sexual violence programs can be seen in the objectives outlined in the Appendix.

Given the similarity in objectives, it is not surprising that evaluations of these prevention programs present similar findings. That is, nearly all of the programs appear to be successful in changing adolescents' and young adults' attitudes about dating (Avery-Leaf et al., 1997; Foshee et al., 2000; Jaffe et al., 1992; Lavoie et al., 1995; Macgowan, 1997; Jones, 1991; Krajewski et al., 1996; Weisz & Black, 2001; Wekerle & Wolfe, 1998) and sexual violence (Anderson et al., 1998; Black et al., 2000; Dallager & Rosén, 1993; Earle, 1996; Ellis, O'Sullivan, & Sowards, 1992; Feltey, Ainslie, & Geib; 1991; Fonow et al., 1992; Foubert, 2000; Foubert & Marriott, 1997; Foubert & McEwen, 1998; Frazier et al., 1994; Gilbert, Heesacker, & Gannon, 1991; Gray et al., 1990; Harrison et al., 1991; Heppner et al., 1999; Heppner, Good et al., 1995; Heppner, Humphrey et al., 1995; Holcomb, Sarvela, Sondag, & Holcomb, 1993; Lanier et al., 1998; Lenihan et al., 1992; Lonsway et al., 1998; Lonsway & Kothari, 2000; Patton & Mannison, 1993; Pinzone-Glover et al., 1998; Rosenthal et al., 1995; Schewe & O'Donohue, 1993, 1996) in the desired direction. The only dating violence program that failed to demonstrate change in high school students' attitudes toward the use of dating violence was Levy's (1984, as cited by Avery-Leaf et al., 1997) Skills for Violence Free Relationships, but it is speculated that changes in attitudes may not have been adequately captured as a result of restricted ranges in measurement. Only 8 of the 40 sexual assault prevention programs failed to demonstrate change in college students' attitudes toward rape (Berg, Lonsway, & Fitzgerald, 1999; Breitenbecher & Scarce, 2001; Gidycz, Layman et al., 2001; Gidycz, Lynn et al., 2001; Heppner, Humphrey et al., 1995; Linz et al., 1990; Nelson & Torgler, 1990; Schaeffer & Nelson, 1993). It should, however, be noted that although Gidycz, Layman, and colleagues' (2001) program did not significantly affect attitudes toward women or rape, it was successful at decreasing rape myth acceptance.

Most programs also show increased knowledge about dating and sexual violence and about the myths that surround partner abuse (Foshee et al., 2000; Jaffe et al., 1992; Jones, 1991; Krajewski et al., 1996; Lavoie et al., 1995; Macgowan, 1997; Weisz & Black, 2001; Wolfe et al., 1996) and sexual assault (Breitenbecher & Scarce, 1999; Hanson & Gidycz,

1993; Heppner, Humphrey et al., 1995; Himelein, 1999; Lonsway & Kothari, 2000; Pinzone-Glover et al., 1998). Six studies report significant positive changes in behavioral intention in hypothetical conflict situations as well (Foubert, 2000; Foubert & Marriott, 1997; Foubert & McEwen, 1998; Gray et al., 1990; Jaffe et al., 1992; Schewe & O'Donohue, 1996). Thus, the majority of dating and sexual violence prevention programs are effective at changing attitudes in a positive direction and at increasing participants' knowledge about dating and sexual violence issues.

EVIDENCE FOR REDUCTIONS IN RATES OF VIOLENCE PERPETRATION AND VICTIMIZATION

In terms of behavioral change among dating violence prevention programs, two of the three programs that assessed behavioral change report that their interventions were effective in reducing the frequency of perpetration of dating violence. At the one-month follow-up of the Safe Dates Project, a universal prevention program, perpetration rates of both psychological and physical abuse were significantly lower among adolescents in the intervention condition in comparison to those of adolescents in the control condition (Foshee, 1998). However, by the one-year follow-up these differences were no longer significant (Foshee et al., 2000). Also of importance is the fact that no significant changes in victimization rates were reported at either the one-month or the one-year follow-up. That is, the Safe Dates Project did not appear to significantly impact victimization rates.

Using growth curve modeling, Wolfe and colleagues (2003) also found both perpetration of physical abuse as well as the use of threatening behaviors to significantly decrease across time in a population targeted for being high-risk for interpersonal violence (i.e., students with a history of childhood maltreatment recruited from Child Protection Services agencies). Although their data reveal a decrease for both intervention and control participants, the slope of the decrease in aggression and threatening behaviors was steeper for adolescents in the intervention condition than for adolescents in the control condition. This same pattern of findings also applied to victimization rates. That is, Wolfe and colleagues reported a significant decrease in victimization rates across time for both intervention and control participants, with a steeper decrease for the intervention group. Thus, findings from these two studies fortunately provide evidence suggesting that dating violence prevention programs can be successful at reducing perpetration and possibly victimization rates, although it is not known how long lasting these effects might prove to be. Further research is nonetheless needed to confirm these findings, and to examine the long-term utility of the programs.

Interestingly, the two dating violence programs that demonstrate positive behavioral change in addition to positive attitudinal change and increases in knowledge about dating violence also prove to be two of the longest interventions. While the majority of the adolescent dating violence prevention programs consist of approximately one to five sessions, the Safe Dates Project (Foshee et al., 1996) includes ten 45-minute sessions and the Youth Relationships Project (Wolfe et al., 1996) consists of eighteen 120-minute sessions. Although it is intuitive that programs aimed at changing behaviors in addition to attitudes would most likely be longer than programs aimed solely at changing attitudes, no data exist as to how much longer interventions need to be in order to demonstrate behavioral effects. In addition, it is not known how much more extensive targeted programs need to be than universal programs in order to produce positive behavioral and attitudinal changes.

In terms of the results of behavioral change among the sexual assault prevention programs, only three programs significantly reduced sexual assault victimization rates (Gidycz, Lynn et al., 2001; Hanson & Gidycz, 1993; Marx et al., 2001). Hanson and Gidycz demonstrated a statistically significant decrease in the rates of sexual assault victimization over a 9-week period among college women with no prior history of sexual victimization. Marx and colleagues similarly found that while 30% of women with a history of sexual victimization in the control condition were raped within two months of the pretest assessment, only 12% of women in the treatment condition reported being raped during this same period. Likewise, in their evaluation of a three-hour didactic intervention implemented with women, Gidycz, Lynn, and colleagues found the following interaction: of the women who had experienced sexual victimizations other than rape during the two-month follow-up period, women in the treatment condition were significantly less likely to have been sexually assaulted during the six-month follow-up period than were women in the control group.

In contrast, sexual assault prevention programs implemented by Breitenbecher and Gidycz (1998), Breitenbecher and Scarce (1999, 2001), Foubert (2000), and Gidycz, Layman, and colleagues (2001) were not successful at reducing the incidence of sexual assault. Taken together, these findings present mixed evidence for the effectiveness of sexual assault programs in reducing victimization.

Inconsistent findings also emerge among studies that evaluate the effectiveness of sexual assault programs in reducing risky dating behaviors (e.g., consuming alcohol or other drugs, isolation of incident site, and the male initiating and paying all the expenses of a date). For instance, although Hanson and Gidycz's (1993) and Himelein's (1999) sexual assault programs led to decreases in risky dating behaviors, evaluations of Breitenbecher and Gidycz's (1998), Breitenbecher and Scarce's (2001), and Gidycz, Lynn et al.'s (2001) programs did not.

Only two programs were found to significantly reduce the likelihood of sexual assault perpetration (Linz et al., 1990; Schewe & O'Donohue, 1993). Linz and colleagues found educational interventions designed to mitigate the effects of media portrayals of violence against women to significantly reduce male college students' sexually coercive behaviors. Schewe and O'Donohue similarly demonstrated that an empathy-facilitating program was successful at significantly reducing the likelihood of engaging in sexual abuse, sexual harassment, and rape in a sample of men who were deemed high-risk for perpetrating sexual aggression. Reductions in perpetration rates were not, however, found by Foubert (2000) and Gidycz, Layman, and colleagues (2001). Evidence for the effectiveness of sexual assault prevention programs in reducing perpetration therefore remains mixed.

Summary of Dating and Sexual Violence Prevention Programs

In summary, based on the few dating violence and sexual assault prevention programs that have been evaluated and published to date, it appears as though such programs are quite successful at changing attitudes and increasing knowledge about physical and sexual partner violence. Moreover, there is some evidence to suggest that a handful of these programs are also successful at reducing rates of dating violence perpetration, and possibly dating violence victimization as well. There is less evidence to suggest that sexual assault prevention programs are successful at initiating behavioral change, largely due to the lack of evaluation of the effectiveness of sexual assault prevention programs in reducing perpetration rates. Studies evaluating the effectiveness of sexual assault prevention programs in reducing victimization rates are similarly inconclusive.

LIMITATIONS TO EXISTING
VIOLENCE PREVENTION PROGRAMS

Several concerns exist within the dating and sexual violence prevention literature.

Ceiling Effects

As Wekerle and Wolfe (1999) warn, "attitudinal measurement is limited by a ceiling effect, because the majority of youth in low-risk samples possess reasonable attitudes about more extreme forms of dating and marital violence at pretest" (p. 448). Ceiling effects were apparent in at least two of the dating violence studies (Avery-Leaf et al., 1997; Jaffe et al, 1992) and in several of the sexual assault studies, especially those that included females in their samples (e.g., Heppner, Humphrey, et al., 1995; Lanier et al., 1998). There is a long established finding that women tend to score in the more desirable direction in comparison to their male counterparts on various knowledge and attitudinal measures related to sexual aggression (e.g., Harrison et al., 1991; Nelson & Torgler, 1990). Given this fact, there is often little room for more desirable change. Use of high-risk samples such as Wolfe and colleagues' (2003) sample of adolescents with a childhood history of maltreatment is one way of avoiding ceiling effects. However, there are also advantages to implementing prevention programs in general samples in that a wide, cross-section of individuals are reached. Despite these advantages, the concern of possible ceiling effects still exists.

Lack of Demonstrated Change in Behavior

As stated above, only two of the dating violence studies show that intervention participants report less perpetration of dating violence than control participants (Foshee et al., 2000; Wolfe et al., 2003), and only one of these studies also report significant changes in victimization rates (Wolfe et al., 2003). Similarly, only three sexual assault prevention programs demonstrate statistically significant decreases in rates of sexual assault victimization (Gidycz, Lynn et al., 2001; Hanson & Gidycz, 1993; Marx et al., 2001), and only two (Linz et al., 1990; Schewe & O'Donohue, 1993) demonstrate statistically significant decreases in the likelihood of sexual assault perpetration. Thus, further research is necessary to develop components that will result in positive behavioral change.

Prevention programs need to focus more intensively on behavioral rather than just attitudinal change, and might benefit from the use of more role-playing and modeling exercises. Furthermore, program developers should be particularly concerned with developing prevention programs that will produce positive changes in both victimization and perpetration rates.

It is also suggested that evaluations of programs include more behaviorally focused measures. Three of the dating violence studies and nine of the sexual assault studies reviewed in this paper included some measure of behavioral change. The most common measure, used by eight of the programs (Breitenbecher & Gidycz, 1998; Breitenbecher & Scarce, 1999, 2001; Foubert, 2000; Gidycz, Layman et al., 2001; Gidycz, Lynn et al., 2001; Hanson & Gidycz, 1993; Marx et al., 2001) was the Sexual Experiences Survey (SES; Koss & Gidycz, 1985). Avery-Leaf et al. (1997) and Foshee et al. (2000) used modified versions of the Conflict Tactics Scale (CTS; Straus, 1979) to collect dating violence perpetration and victimization rates. Wolfe et al. (2003) attempted a multi-method, multi-respondent evaluation design, which included the use of questionnaires, interviews, videotaped observations, audiotape coding, and data collected from participants' dating partners, parents, same sex peers, and teachers as well as from Child Protective Services social workers. However, they reported that they were not able to collect highly informative data from participants' parents, teachers, peers, or dating partners due to either a lack of respondents' knowledge about the participants' dating relationships or a lack of desire to participate. Despite these methodological difficulties, subsequent research using multi-method (interview and self-report), multi-respondent (self and partner) evaluations should be attempted and implemented whenever possible.

Need for Long-Term Follow-Ups

Most of the findings that have been reported on the effectiveness of dating violence and sexual assault prevention programs are based on follow-up data that only extend a few months past the completion of the program. Again, only two dating violence studies (Foshee et al., 2000; Wekerle & Wolfe, 1998) include longer follow-ups (e.g., over 12 months). Foshee et al.'s one-year follow-up data suggest that while cognitive risk factor effects were maintained, behavioral effects were beginning to fade. Data collected by Wolfe and colleagues (1996) beyond the 16-month follow-up have not yet been published. Similarly, programs within the sexual assault literature typically possess follow-ups of only one to seven months, with the exception of one evaluation which extended two years (Lonsway et al., 1998). More importantly, of the sexual assault studies that did include follow-up assessments, seven of them found rebound effects in attitudes (Anderson et al., 1998; Foubert & Marriott, 1997; Frazier et al., 1994; Heppner, Good et al., 1995; Heppner, Humphrey et al., 1995; Heppner et al., 1999; Lonsway & Kothari, 2000). Thus, future research is needed to gain a better understanding of the long-term effects of dating and sexual violence prevention programs.

Furthermore, future research is needed to determine whether attitudinal changes eventually lead to behavioral changes. We do not know how the changes in adolescents' or young adults' attitudes and knowledge about dating and sexual violence come into play when/if they are actually confronted with incidents of dating or sexual violence. In addition, given that there is evidence to suggest that attitudes are likely to fade, investigations should be undertaken to determine whether booster sessions are necessary and whether such sessions would augment the positive effects that are found in attitudinal and knowledge changes.

Lack of Dismantling Studies

None of the dating aggression and few of the sexual aggression programs evaluated separate components within their overall programs. Therefore, little is known about which modules of the interventions are most effective and thus essential, which modules may be less efficacious and in need of improvement, or which components possess no existing benefit and should be discarded. Similarly, very little is known about whether there are components that actually impeded the interventions, or whether there are certain components that appear redundant. In addition, there is little data available to test whether there were additive or interactional effects among components. Research focused on testing the effectiveness of specific components within interventions is thus needed. Such endeavors can aid in the construction of maximally effective interventions.

Reliance on Self-Report Measures

Outside of Wolfe et al.'s (1996) Youth Relationships Project, all other evaluations were based exclusively on self-report data. As a result, there is no corroboration of participants' reports. Information collected from participants' partners would likely prove useful in understanding and documenting the effects of the dating and sexual violence prevention programs. For instance, one possible reason that Foshee (1998) found significant changes in the desired direction in perpetration rates from pretest to the one-month follow-up, but did not also find significant changes in victimization rates is that both partners of a couple were not necessarily in the intervention condition (or program) together. In fact, Foshee and colleagues (2000) report that 75% of the girls in their sample were dating boys older than the boys in the sample and 75% of the boys in their sample were dating girls younger than the girls in the sample. Thus, although perpetration rates among participants in the intervention may have declined, victimization rates for participants who were dating violent, non-participant partners may have remained high. By collecting data from participants' partners, such patterns could be accounted for and documented. This is just one illustration of the advantages of collecting multiple forms of data from a variety of respondents. Future research should investigate whether prevention programs are more effective when both members of the couple participate in the program rather than when only one partner participates.

Comparisons of Universal and Targeted Prevention Programs

Another gap in the literature proves to be a comparison of the effectiveness of universal versus targeted prevention programs for dating and sexual violence. Only six programs targeted at reducing interpersonal violence within high-risk samples exist within these two literatures (five sexual assault programs and one dating violence program; Breitenbecher & Gidycz, 1998; Frazier et al., 1994; Marx et al., 2001; Schewe & O'Donohue, 1993, 1996; Wolfe et al., 1996). Thus, future research should focus on individuals at high risk for dating and sexual violence. In addition, as the field develops, meta-analytic reviews will need to be conducted in order to summarize the overall effectiveness of universal and targeted programs. Results of such studies would prove essential in informing the field as to what direction future prevention efforts should take.

Summary

In summary, several concerns arise from the evaluations of published dating and sexual violence prevention programs. These concerns include difficulties in interpreting results of the effects of such prevention programs as a result of possible ceiling effects and infrequent use of behaviorally focused measures. In addition, the lack of such factors as long-term follow-ups, evaluations of specific components within interventions, corroborating reports from others, and meta-analytic reviews of universal programs and programs targeted for individuals at high risk for dating and sexual violence also impede full evaluation of such programs. As a result of these concerns and the relatively small number of evaluations of dating and sexual violence prevention programs, we also review other related prevention literatures, including prevention programs aimed at reducing delinquent behavior and substance abuse.

PREVENTION OF DELINQUENT BEHAVIOR AND SUBSTANCE USE

The developmental period spanning adolescence and early adulthood is one in which transitions to adult roles often correspond with the initiation or increase of a variety of potentially harmful behaviors, including violence and aggression against peers, as well as alcohol, tobacco, and illicit drug use (Hamburg, 1997). These behaviors pose both current risks (i.e., drunk driving, delinquency) and detrimental long-term outcomes (i.e., substance addiction). In contrast to dating violence, a multitude of prevention efforts have been designed to target these delinquent and antisocial behaviors with the goal of preventing or reducing their occurrence. While some programs primarily target the family and community environments, as with dating violence, many others focus on intact units such as school or college settings as a way to introduce prevention concepts (e.g., Walter, 2001). Unit-based programs may be particularly well suited to prevention efforts, because the programs reach a large cross-section of young adults and provide a format for group-level instruction.

For instance, due to concerns about unacceptably high levels of violence on school campuses, several prevention programs have been designed and implemented to reduce the occurrence of aggressive tactics in conflict resolution. Although prevention programs are recommended for college populations (e.g., LaVant, 2001), most work in this area has focused on elementary through adolescent ages. While many programs have not received empirical evaluation, or lack characteristics such as random assignment that are essential to full program evaluation, we will briefly summarize the existing information on program evaluation from 1990 to the present in this field and then draw conclusions about what programs appear most useful (and least useful) at reducing violent behavior in school settings. We will also review the design, implementation, and success of prevention efforts targeting a range of other antisocial behaviors in young adulthood within the last decade, primarily in the area of substance use.

We will begin with a brief overview of the overall effectiveness of prevention programs targeting antisocial and delinquent behaviors, with an emphasis on overall effectiveness. Then we will discuss a variety of program and research design issues that can be used to maximize the effectiveness of prevention programs in general. We reiterate that we are reviewing the research on prevention of delinquency and substance abuse because there have been many more evaluations of such programs compared to prevention of physical aggression against intimate partners, and because lessons learned from these endeavors may help us design more effective partner violence prevention programs.

OVERALL EFFECTIVENESS OF PREVENTION PROGRAMS

Over the last decade, several exhaustive meta-analyses of prevention programs have helped shed light on the magnitude of change to be expected in various program formats. Using criteria developed by Cohen (1969), the effect size statistic (ES) is a standardized indicator of the effect of treatment compared to control that is independent of sample size and is computed as the difference between the two treatment means divided by the pooled standard deviation. The magnitude of the ES (.20 = small, .50 = medium, .80 = large) is an indication of the number of standard deviation units a person (or group of people) can be expected to improve as a result of treatment.

In an early evaluation of 40 universal prevention programs, Baker, Swisher, Nadenichek, and Popowicz (1984) reported an average effect size (ES) of .55 (with outliers removed) across a wide range of universal prevention studies targeting elementary through college-aged students. The ES of .55 is considered a medium effect size according to Cohen (1969). Specific prevention strategies varied in effectiveness, with an ES of .26 (small effect) for interventions targeted to improving cognitive coping skills and an ES of .93 (large effect; with outliers removed) for interventions focused on communication coping skills.

Lipsey (1992), in a meta-analytic review of predominantly targeted prevention programs for delinquent behavior, demonstrated an average ES across 397 studies to be .17, a small effect. In contrast, Lipsey and Wilson (1993) reported an average effect size for 156 meta-analytic reviews of 9,400 interventions across the social and behavioral sciences of .47, nearly a medium effect size. Thus, it appears that dysfunctional or delinquent behavior may be particularly difficult to change compared to other types of problematic functioning. However, as will be discussed below, the seriousness of the outcomes of youth delinquency may warrant the use of prevention efforts with small effect sizes.

In the most comprehensive meta-analysis of school-based prevention programs to date, Wilson, Gottfredson, and Najaka (2001) examined the effect sizes of 165 studies targeted toward the prevention of crime, substance use, dropout/nonattendance, and related conduct problems. Results confirm previous summaries of the literature and indicate that, while effect sizes are small, the most effective programs are social skills based, with cognitive-behavioral or behavioral instruction (ESs range from .05 to .22). Negative effects were found for other counseling techniques, including non-cognitive-behavioral counseling and social work (ESs range from −.18 to −.14). Concordant with previous investigations, targeted prevention programs demonstrated greater effectiveness (ES = .20) than universal prevention programs (ES = .07).

Similar trends in effectiveness have been found in evaluation of programs specifically targeting alcohol use. In an evaluation of 15 targeted prevention programs for college students, Walters and Bennett (2000) determined that a range of attitudinal and skills-based approaches showed consistently modest effects, whereas purely educational interventions were the least effective. Further, Walters, Bennett, and Noto (2000) recommend that preventions efforts for college students alter attitudes towards alcohol, enhance social problem solving, and provide personalized feedback using norm comparisons rather than providing didactic information on risks.

Prevention Program Design Issues

Universal versus Targeted Prevention Programs. Efficacy differences between universal and targeted intervention efforts typically indicate greater effects for targeted interventions, which are generally more intensive and focused and have a greater ability to detect reductions in destructive behavior due to higher rates of overall frequency of occurrence. Wilson et al. (2001) reported small effect sizes for targeted prevention programs (ES = .20) and even smaller for universal prevention programs (ES = .07). Further, Guerra, Tolan, and Hammond (1994), in a review of universal violence prevention in the schools, argue that while universal interventions may have some utility in changing norms for inappropriate behavior, reducing violent acts, and preventing intermittent violence, they often have little effect in reducing aggressive behavior in chronically violent youth. Thus, they recommend targeted prevention programs for at-risk individuals that use a combination of validated techniques to change the affective, cognitive, and behavioral repertoire of individuals prone to aggression.

An example of the differential effects of universal versus targeted intervention is a program reported by Hausman, Pierce, and Briggs (1996). The study consisted of a multi-component violence prevention program evaluated with 10th graders in three Boston high schools over a period of three years. Using non-random assignment by schools matched for demographic similarity, the project compared: (a) the Violence Prevention Curriculum for Adolescents and the Violence Prevention Project, two components of a school-wide universal violence reduction program; (b) the Fenway Project, an intensive in-class targeted prevention program; and (c) a comparison school with no violence prevention programs in place.

In the school-wide exposure group (n = 331), the Violence Prevention Curriculum consisted of mandatory health class instruction for all 10th graders consisting of education regarding the risk factors contributing to violence and behavioral alternatives to physical conflict. Schools in this group were also exposed to the Violence Prevention Project, which included school-wide presentations on violence prevention and services responding to homicides within the school. In the Fenway Project group, a small number of high-risk students (n = 61) were referred by school staff and enrolled in small classes with higher teacher to student ratios and greater attention to supportiveness and parent involvement. These students were also exposed to the Violence Prevention Curriculum for Adolescents, whereas the remainder of their school was not. Finally, students at the non-exposed school (n = 351) were intended to receive no violence prevention instruction, although the authors discovered that one of the three cohorts of sophomores did in fact receive the Violence Prevention Curriculum, limiting the status of that cohort as a control.

Evaluation of this program targeted change in suspension rates between sophomore and junior years. Although only 50% of suspension rates were due to direct violent episodes (i.e., violent behavior, weapons carrying, and disturbances), the authors reasoned that other high-risk behaviors (i.e., substance use, theft, and sexual harassment) should also be assessed as possible outcomes of a social intervention. Results demonstrated that the in-class exposed group showed a statistically significant reduction in suspension rates during the junior year, with non-exposed students in the same school being 3.7 times more likely to be suspended after controlling for baseline characteristics of the groups. In contrast, the school-wide exposure group showed trends toward less suspension, although the rates were non-significant. Finally, the non-exposed school demonstrated fairly consistent levels of suspension across the sophomore and junior years, with the exception of one year in which suspensions significantly increased.

Thus, the results of this study emphasize that the in-class, targeted intervention was more effective at reducing suspension rates for antisocial behaviors than school-wide universal prevention efforts. However, the broad focus of the targeted prevention program, which included elements beyond violence prevention, as well as the broad definition of the outcome measure as all suspensions regardless of aggression, indicates that this result may reflect better overall school and social adjustment rather than actual reduction in violent behavior. Further, because of the lack of random assignment, as well as the contamination of the comparison school, an evaluation of the school-wide intervention is tentative at best. Thus, this program illustrates several design issues to be discussed later that should be taken into account when implementing prevention programs.

Didactic Instruction versus Interactive Techniques. Over time, the utility of interactive techniques such as role playing, discussion, and behavioral rehearsal has been identified through reviews and meta-analyses as a critical element in maintaining participant attention and in providing experiential learning during the acquisition of new skills (e.g., Dusenbury, Falco, Lake, Brannigan, & Bosworth, 1997). Didactic teaching methods or scare tactics that seek to increase the individual's knowledge of the effects and risks of the problematic behavior are less effective (Gottfredson, 1997; Walters, Bennett, & Noto, 2000). For instance, Lipsey (1992) reported a negative ES ($-.24$) for programs such as shock incarceration and "scared straight" methods that utilize fear of negative consequences as a motivator for change. Similarly, Walters and Bennett (2000) determined that a range of attitudinal and skills-based approaches show consistently positive albeit small effects in preventing drinking in college students, whereas purely educational interventions generally are not effective.

Further, Tobler and Stratton (1997), in a meta-analysis of 120 drug prevention programs, concluded that programs employing interactive techniques were more effective than those that did not. The authors also concluded that the considerable association between delivery technique (interactive vs. non-interactive) and content of the program (social influence, informational, affective) indicated that interactive delivery might explain the greater effectiveness of certain program types.

The failure of didactic instruction to change behavior is particularly apparent in two recent published reports of universal prevention efforts to reduce tobacco use by adolescents. Aveyard et al. (2001) reported the results of a randomized prevention and cessation program for over 8,000 British adolescents (13-14 yrs.). The intervention consisted of three class sessions and three computer sessions that provided information about the stages of change, the consequences of smoking, facts about smoking, and a personal assessment of the current stage of change and method for moving to the next stage. Results of the intervention indicated no significant effect on either stage of change or smoking status.

Similarly, Hancock, Sanson-Fisher, Perkins, Girgis, Howley, and Schofield (2001) reported no significant effects for a broad-based community intervention for over 3,000 rural Australian adolescents that attempted to increase awareness of smoking risk and promote community involvement for tobacco cessation. In contrast, Sussman, Lichtman, Ritt, and Pallonen (1999) reported that, of 17 universal tobacco prevention programs that included attention to normative and/or informational social influence variables, there was a modest mean difference in tobacco use between intervention and control conditions of 6%, indicating that a focus on changing cognitions regarding tobacco use and equipping individuals with skills to resist pressure to smoke demonstrates more utility that didactic instruction regarding risk factors.

Perhaps the most well known prevention failure is the widely implemented drug use prevention program, DARE (Drug Awareness Resistance Education). Using primarily didactic instruction techniques presented by uniformed law enforcement officers, DARE has been implemented with thousands of elementary through high school age students across the United States. However, Gottfredson (1997) reported that empirical evaluations consistently demonstrate little to no change in outcome. For example, Clayton, Cattarello, and Johnstone (1996) reported short-term and four-year follow-up results for 2000 students indicating that, while there were some short-term changes in attitudes toward drug use, these did not persist over time. Further, there was no significant effect for change in drug use behavior at any time point. Similarly, Lynam et al. (1999) reported very few significant effects on attitude or behavior for 1,000 students at 10-years post-intervention.

To summarize, Gottfredson (1997), in a comprehensive review of 149 published studies of school-based prevention studies, concluded that the bulk of evidence to date suggests that for both delinquency and substance use in school-aged individuals, instructional programs are ineffective at reducing problem behaviors. Thus, focusing exclusively on fear tactics, information and risk factors, or moral appeals has little to no significant effect on the targeted behaviors. Conversely, Gottfredson reported the greatest success for universal prevention programs in two areas: norm-based education and social skills programs. Norm-based programs typically include procedures designed to provide clear rules with consistent enforcement and group-level transmittal of behavioral norms through campaigns or ceremonies. Social skills programs can encompass a variety of procedures designed to increase individual efficacy in conflictual social interactions (i.e., communication and problem-solving) and typically require long time periods (i.e., multi-year) to successfully reinforce skills. Further, Gottfredson concluded that behavior modification programs for at-risk individuals are most effective at reducing substance use in youth.

Cognitive-Behavioral versus Non-Cognitive Behavioral Treatment Orientation. Several reviews and meta-analyses converge in their finding that behavioral or cognitive-behavioral programs demonstrate greater efficacy than non-cognitive behavioral programs. For instance, Walters et al. (2000), in a review of college alcohol use prevention programs, recommend that preventions efforts alter attitudes towards alcohol, enhance social problem solving, and provide personalized feedback using norm comparisons rather than providing didactic information on risks or using abstinence based approaches. Similarly, in the most comprehensive meta-analysis of school-based prevention programs to date, Wilson et al. (2001) examined the effect sizes of 165 studies targeted toward the prevention of crime, substance use, dropout/nonattendance, and related conduct problems. Results indicate that, while effect sizes are small, the most effective programs are social skills based, with cognitive-behavioral or behavioral instruction (ESs range from .05 to .22). Negative effects were found for other counseling techniques, including non-cognitive-behavioral counseling and social work (ESs range from −.18 to −.14).

Thus, the most successful universal and targeted prevention efforts involve the use of behavioral and cognitive-behavioral strategies intended to alter beliefs, attributions, and responses to situations in which problematic behavior currently exists. We will now provide a brief summary of two empirically validated strategies. First, the goal of *social skills training* is to increase the likelihood of healthy choices in situations involving conflict or pressure to engage in a dangerous activity; individuals are trained how to think of alternative responses to problematic situations, how to evaluate consequences of each possible action, and how to implement the chosen solution (Gottfredson, 1997). For instance, Huesmann and colleagues (1996) describe the development of a violence prevention program for urban schools that attempts to alter individual's beliefs and actions. Through a combined universal and targeted approach, a program was implemented to increase motivation to behave in socially appropriate ways, to decrease acceptance of violent solutions to conflict, and to improve cognitive and behavioral repertoires in dealing with conflictual situations.

Second, based on the concepts that (a) individuals often overestimate the frequency of problem behaviors among their peers and that (b) these behaviors are often considered acceptable among at least a minority of individuals within a given group, *norms-based education* attempts to make explicit appropriate norms for behavior. Activities include clarifying rules for appropriate behavior, enforcing discipline upon rule violation, and announcements, ceremonies, and symbols intended to remind individuals about appropriate behavior (Gottfredson, 1997). Wynn, Schulenberg, Maggs, and Zucker (2000), for instance, reported findings from a school-based universal prevention program for alcohol use that included training in both refusal skills and norm setting as part of a larger intervention. While both refusal skills and awareness of drinking norms improved as a result of the program, only norm setting mediated the effect of the intervention on alcohol overindulgence. Further, norm setting was only a significant mediator for older students (7th to 8th and 8th to 10th grade intervals) versus younger students (6th to 7th grade interval), indicating that normative comparisons may be more developmentally appropriate for older adolescents.

Some evidence also indicates that providing feedback contrasting individual behavior to norms for the population results in decreased problem behavior, presumably because individuals are unaware that their behavior deviates from the norm. The approach is similar to the short motivational interview used to reduce drinking in alcoholics (Miller, 1989). For example, Marlatt et al. (1998) implemented a targeted prevention program with 348 college freshman at high-risk for binge drinking using a brief format that included assessment, individualized feedback, and advice. Results demonstrated significant decreases in binge drinking over time compared to a no-treatment control group, with standardized ESs ranging from .15 for the 6-month follow-up of frequency and quantity of alcohol consumption to .32 for the two-year follow-up of alcohol-related problems. Thus, norm-based approaches appear promising for reducing drinking in less severe populations, and may be particularly helpful in reducing the negative consequences (i.e., social and occupational problems) associated with excessive drinking.

Treatment Dosage. The length and extensiveness of prevention programs may be related to both short-term change as well as long-term maintenance of change. Lipsey (1992), for instance, reported that greater dosages of treatment for juvenile delinquents (as a composite of treatment duration, frequency of contact, and total hours of contact) yielded larger effect sizes than more minimal programs. An excellent example of both short-term change and long-term attenuation of change comes from outcome reports of Project Northland, an extensive multi-component universal prevention program targeting alcohol use in middle-school adolescents (Perry et al., 1996). The program consisted of a three-year intervention with cognitive-behavioral in-class training, peer leadership, parental involvement, and community task forces. While short-term results appeared promising, and indicated significant reductions in self-reports of drinking, significant effects disappeared by the two-year follow-up. The researchers then decided to implement a developmentally appropriate "phase 2" prevention program targeting late high school students by altering community norms about appropriate alcohol use (Williams & Perry, 1998). Thus, even extensive universal prevention programs that demonstrate short-term efficacy may require repeated implementation to achieve long-term desired results.

Cultural Awareness. Sensitivity to different ethnic and cultural backgrounds has also been posited as an important consideration in program development (e.g., Dusenbury et al., 1997). Yung and Hammond (1998) report on a targeted intervention program designed for African-American youth that includes social skills training, anger management training, and violence education with an emphasis on cultural sensitivity and avoidance of stigmatization. While the program design is based on existing principles of prevention, elements such as the use of ethnically similar role models, ethnically congruent language, and ethnically relevant program content are included to ensure that the program resonates with the population being targeted. The evaluation of the program is compromised by lack of both random assignment and tests of statistical significance, but the authors reported that on average the ratio of violent and other criminal offensives between the prevention and control groups was about 1:2, indicating that the program may be effective at reducing aggressive behavior in African-American youth.

Prevention Research Design Issues

Assignment to Treatment. Many outcome evaluations of prevention programs lack appropriate random assignment to conditions, which limits the validity of the findings. Assignment to conditions based on availability of the individuals, motivation and ability of the educators, or other biased factors precludes generalizability to populations in which less than ideal circumstances exist. Further, because many problematic behaviors naturally increase in frequency over time due to developmental maturation, lack of a proper control group limits the ability to examine differences between prevention programs and the course of a behavior without intervention (e.g., Miller, Toscova, Miller, & Sanchez, 2000). Finally, results from meta-analysis indicate that random assignment to condition was associated with effect sizes three times as large (ES = .25) as non-random assignment (ES = .08; Wilson et al., 2001) in studies of prevention of school based problem behaviors like aggression and substance abuse.

The importance of random assignment is demonstrated by the evaluation of the Students for Peace project (Orpinas, Kelder, Frankowski, Murray, Zhang, & McAlister, 2000), which in its final form consisted of an intensive, multifaceted universal prevention program for adolescents. Procedures included developing a school health promotion council, instituting "Second Step: A Violence Prevention Curriculum" (Committee for Children, 1990), implementing peer mediation and counseling programs, and educating parents. The Second Step program included violence education, and training in empathy, conflict resolution, and anger management. A small pilot project of the program ($n = 223$; Orpinas, Parcel, McAlister, & Frankowski, 1995) demonstrated some significant effects in reducing self-reported aggression among males. However, the schools were chosen for overall willingness to participate, and highly motivated, competent teachers were selected to implement the program.

When a comprehensive project based on the same program was implemented using random assignment to schools matched on demographic characteristics ($n = 2246$), comparisons yielded no significant effects, with trends opposite the expected direction. The authors attributed their lack of significant effects to high rates of community violence, positive parental attitudes towards using violence to solve problems, difficulties with proper implementation of a multi-component intervention, lack of targeted prevention for high-risk students, and compensatory behaviors by the control schools to implement their own violence prevention initiatives (Orpinas et al., 1995). Thus, while the program appeared promising under ideal conditions, the realities of the inner-city schools in which the program was implemented attenuated the nonrandomized effects. The seemingly positive pre-post results of the initial school based aggression program make sense in that highly motivated teachers participated and the study did not involve a control group. Pre-post interventions without a control group generally yield more positive effects than control group comparisons (Lipsey & Wilson, 1993).

Random Assignment of Individuals versus Groups. An under appreciated problem in prevention research involves the method of analysis often used with school-based interventions. Because it is frequently more feasible to randomly assign intact classrooms or even schools to receive different treatments, individuals within each treatment group are not independent. That is, they share pre-existing characteristics (i.e., neighborhood, school influences) that violate the assumption of independent samples and require allowances for correlated error terms (Kreft, 1997). Examining group-level data at the level of the individual thus often leads to inaccurate effect sizes and imprecise tests for significance (Gottfredson, 1997).

While a solution to the problem of analyzing data from pre-existing intact groups is to conduct all analyses at the level of the randomized group, this is rarely done in prevention research. Wilson et al. (2001), in a meta-analysis of 216 comparisons between interventions and controls, report that while only 32% of studies assigned individuals (versus groups) to treatment, 91% used individual-level analyses to examine their data.

There are two primary reasons for lack of attentiveness to group-level information. First, because such analyses require substantial numbers of groups in each condition, many prevention programs (which often consist of one treatment and one control group) lack adequate power to make distinctions at the group level. Gottfredson (1997) thus argues that funding agencies must allow for studies with adequate numbers of groups to achieve the necessary power to make such comparisons. Second, such aggregated analyses may also be biased because individual-level variability is lost and results are usually inflated or otherwise misleading, thus making inferences about individual reaction to the programs difficult (e.g., Robinson, 1950).

In order to preserve both individual and group level information, one remedy is a nested cross-sectional design with more than one observation for each group that is then analyzed with a Time × Condition mixed model analysis of variance (ANOVA) or covariance (ANCOVA; Murray, Clark, & Wagenaar, 2000). Further, multilevel analysis, in which both individual and group variance is taken into account, can also be an effective solution (Kreft, 1997), particularly when groups differ in their trajectory of change across time.

No Treatment Controls versus Treatment as Usual. Due to federal and local mandates for prevention programs targeting antisocial behavior and substance use, it is to be expected that many of the studies included in the aforementioned meta-analyses and reviews compare prevention programs with control groups receiving treatment as usual (i.e., health classes devoted to substance use education) rather than with groups receiving no treatment. Thus, effect sizes will likely appear smaller for these comparisons, and this is in fact the case (e.g., Lipsey, 1992). The implications for the attenuated effect sizes in studies employing treatment as usual controls are (a) that many current interventions (i.e., health education classes) may be somewhat effective at preventing or reducing the occurrence of deviant behavior and (b) that the small effect sizes witnessed in many of these studies may better represent a lack of improvement over treatment as usual rather than an overall lack of effectiveness for prevention programs in general. Thus, cost-benefit analyses become crucial in deciding whether to implement more extensive, costly programs that may demonstrate little incremental utility over initiatives already in place.

Attitude versus Behavior Change. Particularly in universal prevention research, change in attitudes or knowledge level regarding a specific deviant behavior have been used as an outcome measure of interest under the theory that change in attitude should reflect eventual change in behavior. However, as with the dating violence literature, prevention program evaluations indicate that attitude change does not consistently equate with a change in the problematic behavior of interest (e.g., Walters et al., 2000). Thus, it is essential that behavioral outcomes be assessed in order to demonstrate the true effectiveness of programs aimed at reducing deviant behavior.

Summary of Delinquent Behavior and Substance Use Prevention Programs

Based on the above empirical evaluations, meta-analyses, and reviews of the literature, there is a fair degree of consensus regarding the components of successful prevention designs and research strategies. While effect sizes are often in the small range (ESs of .20 or less), program designs that appear to produce the greatest amount of change share several common features. First, prevention programs targeted towards individuals who are either at higher risk for the development of a deviant behavior, or who are currently displaying low levels of the behavior, tend to produce greater changes (most likely due to the greater variability of the sample). Second, programs that involve interactive components such as role play and discussion consistently demonstrate greater effectiveness than programs based on didactic instruction that simply impart information but do not require participants to actively practice any of the skills taught. Third, treatments with a cognitive or cognitive-behavioral orientation such as social skills training and norms education consistently outperform non-cognitive behavioral programs. Fourth, programs than include scare tactics or threats appear to be contraindicated due to negative effects on outcome. Fifth, longer treatment duration and/or follow-up sessions may produce greater effects than short-term or single time point programs. Sixth, an emphasis on culturally appropriate programs may improve treatment outcome, particularly for social skills based programs, due to the greater likelihood that suggested behavior change will be successful in the individual's environment (although this has yet to be empirically validated).

Similarly, several elements of research design enable more accurate assessments of program effectiveness. First, random assignment to conditions is absolutely essential due to issues of developmental maturation that may mask any effects of treatment. Second, whenever possible it is preferable to randomly assign individuals rather than groups (i.e., classes, units) to treatment groups in order to increase statistical power and decrease the dependence of the sample. Since such assignment often is not feasible, multilevel statistical techniques should be utilized in order to examine both individual- and group-level information. Third, when comparing prevention programs to treatment as usual (e.g., existing health education), small effect sizes may be due to the effectiveness of the "treatment as usual" control group rather than the ineffectiveness of the prevention program. Fourth, due to the lack of correspondence between attitude change and actual change in behavior, outcome measures should rely, at least in part, on assessments of behavior change (i.e., self-report, informant-report, police records).

At a conceptual level, while the effect sizes of many prevention programs are quite small, the above recommendations can help to maximize effectiveness. Further, because these antisocial and delinquent behaviors are destructive in both the immediate sense and in their prediction of long-term problems (i.e., alcoholism, incarceration), improving outcomes for only a minority of participants justifies the expense of many programs.

OVERALL SUMMARY AND CONCLUSIONS

To summarize the dating and sexual violence prevention results, nearly all of the programs increased knowledge about and reduced attitudes supporting dating and sexual aggression. Only 3 of the 9 dating violence studies and 5 of the 40 sexual assault studies provided evaluation of behavioral change. In all three of the dating violence studies that evaluated behavioral change (two universal studies and one targeted intervention), reductions in reports of dating violence perpetration were found. Interestingly, two of the three programs were relatively long in length (ten 45-minute sessions for the universal program and 18 two-hour sessions for the targeted program). Moreover, the 18-session targeted program was the only program to also report decreases in victimization rates. Only two of the sexual assault prevention programs evaluated their effectiveness in reducing perpetration rates, and only three investigated their effectiveness in reducing victimization rates.

Because our review of published dating violence programs yielded only nine controlled outcome studies, we also reviewed related prevention research on delinquency and substance abuse. There is voluminous material on prevention of substance abuse and comparatively less on other forms of delinquent behavior. A primary reason for reviewing the substance abuse and delinquency research was to evaluate the effectiveness of the programs, the successful research designs to address prevention outcomes, and the qualities of successful programs.

Universal prevention programs to reduce varied antisocial behavior like delinquency and substance use aimed at all individuals in a population yield very small effect sizes. Based on meta-analyses, prevention programs targeted to high-risk populations yield somewhat larger, but still relatively small effect sizes. The programs that have the largest effects are those that involve active participation (versus didactic instruction), those that have a cognitive-behavioral orientation (versus non-directive/empathy-oriented programs), and those with greater duration of treatment (i.e., more than one session).

Given the effect sizes obtained in various prevention studies and the magnitude of the problem of partner abuse in young people, a practical approach to addressing partner violence is to provide increasingly intense interventions based on the level of physical aggression present (see Figure 1). Different interventions and different doses or levels of interventions are needed depending upon the frequency and severity of physical aggression. As individuals enter an organization, we recommend that they all receive a universal intervention. For those individuals with moderate levels of aggression, a targeted intervention should be provided, and for those with severe levels of aggression, a more intense targeted intervention may be necessary.

The universal prevention program for all individuals should be the least costly component, with the number of sessions varying from one to several (with a total time of one to five hours). The intervention should be designed to be presented in large groups, and should impart information regarding (a) norms for appropriate behavior and communication techniques in romantic relationships, (b) the risks and negative consequences associated with aggression toward the partner (including harm to the victim and legal repercussions for the perpetrator), and (c) services available to get help if partner aggression occurs (for both the aggressor and the victim).

For individuals with moderate levels of partner aggression, we suggest a targeted intervention of moderate cost and intensity, with sessions of moderate length (with a total time of five to 10 hours). The targeted interventions could involve various components, such as motivational interviewing, social skills and anger management, and relationship therapy. First, small groups of individuals could undergo social skills training classes, in which the lessons introduced in the universal prevention program could be extended and intensified and more individualized attention and feedback could be provided. Second, individual motivational feedback interviews could be conducted to (a) directly contrast the individual's aggression with normative behavior, (b) to assess for awareness of the consequences of such behavior, and (c) to provide individualized recommendations and advice for methods to change. Motivational interviewing could occur in tandem with social skills training, or could be used as a preliminary step before skills training is recommended.

FIGURE 1. Proposed Model of Intimate Partner Violence Prevention

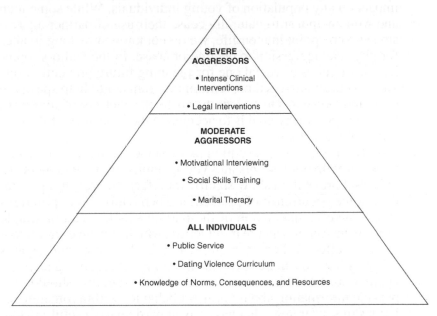

Finally, for those individuals who display persistent and/or severe aggression, mandated interventions should be implemented. These would be longest in duration (with a total time of 15 to 30 hours), and would involve an intensive individualized program based on empirically derived treatment modalities. Because this is not the focus of the current review, however, we will not go into detail about the specific potential components of this intervention.

To summarize, a universal program to reduce or prevent partner aggression has a place in the any population where such a program can be implemented (high school, military, college, police academy, work environments with large numbers of new employees each year) for several reasons:

 a. Some focus on preventing and/or reducing partner aggression has broad scale social and political value and makes clear to the new members that the organization (high school, college, military, academy) will not tolerate partner aggression and that the organization takes partner aggression very seriously.

 b. Young men and women in their late teens to mid twenties are at significantly elevated risk for partner aggression (O'Leary, 1999), and a universal program might thus have significant observable impact on any population of young individuals. While some men and women appear to naturally cease their use of partner aggression at some point in their life, we do not know how long it takes for physical aggression to decline or cease. In the authors' opinion, this issue is a crucial one for planning future prevention services. Thus, a universal prevention program could help speed the cessation process and reduce harm to the victims of abuse. In brief, a very worthy goal is to accelerate the trajectory of the cessation of partner aggression.

c. Based on reviews of prevention of substance abuse and antisocial behavior with adolescents and young adults, two components of universal prevention show significant effects in preventing or reducing the occurrence of problematic behaviors. First, programs should involve interaction of the participants (instead of simple didactic instruction and fear induction, which can have significant negative effects). For example, it is useful to have participants role play how to handle stressful situations without using physical aggression. Second, universal prevention programs should also provide information about norms of behavior within romantic relationships, a strategy that has proven particularly useful in alcohol abuse prevention programs.

In addition to universal prevention programs, a key focus on targeting individuals at moderate risk using more intensive prevention services appears to be warranted for the following reasons:

a. Individuals who have almost no risk for partner aggression may be helped by programs aimed at all individuals (e.g., all college students, all new employees in a large organization, military recruits), but any effects on such individuals will be very hard to document and the cost relative to the benefits will be high.

b. Individuals at very high risk for partner aggression, such as individuals with alcohol problems, a history of physical aggression against peers, or other antisocial behaviors will likely need more than a brief universal prevention program to alter a cluster of problematic behaviors.

c. While programs designed to address all forms of partner violence are warranted (i.e., very low and high risk individuals), the medium risk individuals appear to be the most likely to show change as a result of prevention programs.

Research Recommendations for the Prevention of Intimate Partner Violence

Throughout the above literature review and recommendations for program implementation, we have repeatedly indicated the need for more extensive, well-designed research initiatives to aid in the selection of effective treatments. We now summarize our primary recommendations for future research in this field:

a. Longitudinal studies are sorely needed to ascertain who ceases being physically aggressive against their partners and how soon such cessation begins. Similarly, one should ascertain who escalates from mild to moderate partner aggression and from moderate to severe aggression. The longest published follow-up evaluation of partner aggression in a community sample is only three years (Aldarondo, 1996; Quigley & Leonard, 1996), and thus we desperately need information about the stability and instability of such aggression across time in young men and women in order to more effectively target the individuals at greatest risk for prolonged aggression.

b. Comparing universal and targeted interventions for their relative efficacy in reducing or preventing partner aggression is important both from a cost benefit analysis and from a social policy standpoint.

c. Programs designed to reduce behaviors that co-occur with partner aggression, such as alcohol abuse, conflictual parenting, and relationship discord, may inadvertently help to reduce intimate partner aggression. Evaluation of the value of such programs in preventing partner aggression would be relatively inexpensive and potentially quite valuable. Moreover, given that individuals often voluntarily seek out such programs, the need to persuade aggressive individuals to participate in violence treatments is reduced.

d. Targeting individuals with moderate to severe aggression for intensive programs to reduce and/or prevent escalation to more severe aggression and injury might be especially effective. While there is not unequivocal evidence for the treatment effects of any specific kind of program, there is considerable evidence that partner aggression can be reduced. One main reason for the lack of treatment effects is that individuals in control groups often reduce their behavior as much as those in the treatment groups (e.g., Babcock, Green, & Robie, 2004; Dunford, 2000; Gondolf, 2002). Thus, careful study of the change processes in the control groups (often who get court monitoring or other minimal interventions) is needed.

In conclusion, intimate partner violence prevention programs demonstrate promise in preventing and reducing aggression in young adults. While significant gaps exist in knowledge regarding appropriate program format and targets, the extensive literature on delinquency and substance use prevention programs provide invaluable information regarding the most effective methods for creating and measuring reduction in problematic behavior.

REFERENCES

Aldarondo, E. (1996). Cessation and persistence of wife assault: A longitudinal analysis. *American Journal of Orthopsychiatry, 66*, 141-151.

Anderson, L. A., Stoelb, M. P., Duggan, P., Hieger, B., Kling, K. H., & Payne, J. P. (1998). The effectiveness of two types of rape prevention programs in changing the rape-supportive attitudes of college students. *Journal of College Student Development, 39*, 131-142.

Avery-Leaf, S., Cascardi, M., O'Leary, K. D., & Cano, A. (1997). Efficacy of dating violence prevention program on attitudes justifying aggression. *Journal of Adolescent Health, 21*, 11-17.

Aveyard, P., Sherratt, E., Almond, J., Lawrence, T., Lancashire, R., Griffin, C. et al. (2001). The change-in-stage and updated smoking status results from a cluster-randomized trial of smoking prevention and cessation using the transtheoretical model among British adolescents. *Preventive Medicine, 33*, 313-324.

Babcock, J. C., Green, C. E., & Robie, C. (2004). Does batterers' treatment work? A meta-analytic review of domestic violence treatment. *Clinical Psychology Review, 23*, 1023-1053.

Baker, S. B., Swisher, J. D., Nadenichek, P. E., & Popwicz, C. L. (1984). Measured effects of primary prevention strategies. *Personnel and Guidance Journal, 62*, 459-464.

Berg, D. R., Lonsway, K. A., & Fitzgerald, L. F. (1999). Rape prevention education for men: The effectiveness of empathy-induction techniques. *Journal of College Student Development, 40*, 219-234.

Bird, G. W., Stith, S. M., & Schladale, J. (1991). Psychological resources, coping strategies, and negotiation styles as discriminators of violence in dating relationships. *Family Relation, 40*, 45-50.

Black, B., Weisz, A., Coats, S., & Patterson, D. (2000). Evaluating a psychoeducational sexual assault prevention program incorporating theatrical presentation, peer education, and social work. *Research on Social Work Practice, 10*, 589-606.

Bogal-Allbritten, R. B., & Allbritten, W. L. (1985). The hidden victims: Courtship violence among college students. *Journal of College Student Personnel, 26,* 201-204.

Boyle, D.J., & Vivian, D. (1996). Generalized versus spouse-specific anger/hostility and men's violence against intimates. *Violence and Victims, 11,* 293-317.

Breitenbecher, K. H., & Gidycz, C. A. (1998). An empirical evaluation of a program designed to reduce the risk of multiple sexual victimization. *Journal of Interpersonal Violence, 13,* 472-488.

Breitenbecher, K. H., & Scarce, M. (1999). A longitudinal evaluation of the effectiveness of a sexual assault education program. *Journal of Interpersonal Violence, 14,* 459-478.

Breitenbecher, K. H., & Scarce, M. (2001). An evaluation of the effectiveness of a sexual assault education program focusing on psychological barriers to resistance. *Journal of Interpersonal Violence, 16,* 387-407.

Burcky, W., Reuterman, N., & Kopsky, S. (1988). Dating violence among high school students. *The School Counselor, 35,* 353-358.

Burt, M. R. (1980). Cultural myths and supports for rape. *Journal of Personality and Social Psychology, 38,* 217-230.

Carlson, B. E. (1987). Dating violence: A research review and comparison with spouse abuse. *Social Casework: The Journal of Contemporary Social Work, 68,* 16-23.

Cate, R. M., Henton, J. M., Koval, J., Christopher, F. S., & Lloyd, S. (1982). Premarital abuse: A social psychological perspective. *Journal of Family Issues, 3,* 79-90.

Clayton, R. R., Cattarello, A. M., & Johnstone, B. M. (1996). The effectiveness of Drug Abuse Resistance Education (Project DARE): 5-year follow-up results. *Preventive Medicine, 25,* 307-318.

Cohen, J. (1969). *Statistical power analysis for the behavioral sciences.* New York: Academic Press.

Committee for Children. (1990). *Second Step: A violence prevention curriculum. Grades 6-8.* Seattle, WA: Author.

Dallager, C., & Rosén, L. A. (1993). Effects of a human sexuality course on attitudes toward rape and violence. *Journal of Sex Education and Therapy, 19,* 193-199.

Dobash, R. E., & Dobash, R. P. (1979). *Violence against wives: A case against the patriarchy.* New York: Free Press.

Dunford, F. W. (2000). The San Diego Navy Experiment: An assessment of interventions for men who assault their wives. *Journal of Consulting and Clinical Psychology, 68,* 468-476.

Dusenbury, L., Falco, M., Lake, A., Brannigan, R., & Bosworth, K. (1997). Nine critical elements of promising violence prevention programs. *Journal of School Health, 67,* 409-414.

Dutton, D. G. (1988). *The domestic assault of women: Psychological and criminal justice perspectives.* Boston, MA: Allyn & Bacon.

Earle, J. P. (1996). Acquaintance rape workshops: Their effectiveness in changing the attitudes of first year college men. *National Association of Student Personnel Administrators Journal, 34,* 2-18.

Ellis, A. L., O'Sullivan, C. S., & Sowards, B. A. (1992). The impact of contemplated exposure to a survivor of rape on attitudes toward rape. *Journal of Applied Social Psychology, 22,* 889-895.

Feld, S. L., & Straus, M. A. (1989). Escalation and desistance of violence in marriage. *Criminology, 27,* 141-161.

Feltey, K. M., Ainslie, J. J., & Geib, A. (1991). Sexual coercion attitudes among high school students: The influence of gender and rape education. *Youth & Society, 23,* 229-250.

Finn, J. (1986). The relationship between sex role attitudes and attitudes supporting marital violence. *Sex Roles, 14,* 235-244.

Follingstad, D. R., Wright, S., Lloyd, S., & Sebastian, J. A. (1991). Sex differences in motivations and effects in dating violence. *Family Relations, 40,* 51-57.

Fonow, M. M., Richardson, L., & Wemmerus, V. A. (1992). Feminist rape education: Does it work? *Gender and Society, 6,* 108-121.

Foshee, V. A. (1998). Involving schools and communities in preventing adolescent dating abuse. In X. B. Arriaga & S. Oskamp (Eds.), *Addressing community problems: Psychological research and interventions* (pp. 104-129). Thousand Oaks, CA: Sage Publications, Inc.

Foshee, V. A., Bauman, K. E., Greene, W. F., Koch, G. G., Linder, G. F., & MacDougall, J. E. (2000). The safe dates program: 1-year follow-up results. *American Journal of Public Health, 90,* 1619-1622.

Foshee, V. A., Linder, G. F., Bauman, K., Langwick, S., Arriaga, X., Heath, J. et al. (1996). The Safe Dates project: Theoretical basis, evaluation design, and selected baseline findings. *Journal of Preventative Medicine, 12,* 39-47.

Foubert, J. D. (2000). The longitudinal effects of a rape-prevention program on fraternity men's attitudes, behavioral intent, and behavior. *Journal of American College Health, 48,* 158-163.

Foubert, J. D., & Marriott, K. A. (1997). Effects of a sexual assault peer education program on men's belief in rape myths. *Sex Roles: A Journal of Research, 36,* 259-268.

Foubert, J. D., & McEwen, M. K. (1998). An all-male rape prevention peer education program: Decreasing fraternity men's behavioral intent to rape. *Journal of College Student Development, 39,* 548-556.

Frazier, P., Valtinson, G., & Candell, S. (1994). Evaluation of a coeducational interactive rape prevention program. *Journal of Counseling and Development, 73,* 153-158.

Fritz, P. A. T., & O'Leary, K. D. (2004). Physical and psychological partner aggression across a decade: A growth curve analysis. *Violence and Victims, 19,* 3-16.

Gidycz, C. A., Layman, M. J., Rich, C. L., Crothers, M., Gylys, J., Matorin, A. et al. (2001). An evaluation of an acquaintance rape prevention program: Impact on attitudes, sexual aggression, and sexual victimization. *Journal of Interpersonal Violence, 16,* 1120-1138.

Gidycz, C. A., Lynn, S. J., Rich, C. L., Marioni, N. L., Loh, C., Blackwell, L. et al. (2001). The evaluation of a sexual assault risk reduction program: A multisite investigation. *Journal of Consulting and Clinical Psychology, 69,* 1073-1078.

Gilbert, B. J., Heesacker, M., & Gannon, L. J. (1991). Changing the sexual aggression-supportive attitudes of men: A psychoeducational intervention. *Journal of Counseling Psychology, 38,* 197-203.

Gondolf, E. W. (2002). *Batterer intervention systems: Issues, outcomes, and recommendations.* Thousand Oaks: Sage.

Gottfredson, D. C. (1997). School-based crime prevention. In L. Sherman, D.C. Gottfredson, D. McKenzie, J. Eck, P. Reuter, & S.D. Bushway (Eds.), *Preventing crime: What works, what doesn't, what's promising.* College Park, MD: Department of Criminology and Criminal Justice, University of Maryland. Retrieved January 15, 2002 from, http://www.ncjrs.org/works

Gray, M. D., Lesser, D., Quinn, E., & Bounds, C. (1990). The effectiveness of personalizing acquaintance rape prevention: Programs on perception of vulnerability and on reducing risk-taking behavior. *Journal of College Student Development, 31,* 217-220.

Greenberg, M. T., Domitrovich, C., & Bumbarger, B. (2001, March). The prevention of mental disorders in school-aged children: Current state of the field. *Prevention and Treatment, 4.* Retrieved October 14, 2004 from, http://www.journals.apa.org/prevention

Guerra, N. G., Tolan, P. H., & Hammond, R. (1994). Prevention and treatment of adolescent violence. In L. D. Eron & J. H. Gentry (Eds.), *Reason to hope: A psychosocial perspective on violence and youth* (pp. 383-403). Washington, DC: American Psychological Association.

Hamburg, D. A. (1997). Toward a strategy for healthy adolescent development. *American Journal of Psychiatry, 154,* 7-12.

Hancock, L., Sanson-Fisher, R., Perkins, J., Girgis, A., Howley, P., & Schofield, M. (2001). The effect of a community action intervention on adolescent smoking rates in rural Australian towns: The CART Project. *Preventive Medicine, 32,* 332-340.

Hanson, K. A., & Gidycz, C. A. (1993). Evaluation of a sexual assault prevention program. *Journal of Consulting and Clinical Psychology, 61,* 1046-1052.

Harrison, P. J., Downes, J., & Williams, M. D. (1991). Date and acquaintance rape: Perceptions and attitude change strategies. *Journal of College Student Development, 32,* 131-139.

Hausman, A., Pierce, G., & Briggs, L. (1996). Evaluation of comprehensive violence prevention education: Effects on student behavior. *Journal of Adolescent Health, 19,* 104-110.

Heppner, M. J., Good, G. E., Hillenbrand-Gunn, T. L., Hawkins, A. K., Hacquard, L. L., Nichol, R. K. et al. (1995). Examining sex differences in altering attitudes about rape: A test of the Elaboration Likelihood Model. *Journal of Counseling and Development, 73,* 640-647.

Heppner, M. J., Humphrey, C. F., Hillenbrand-Gunn, T. L., & DeBord, K. A. (1995). The differential effects of rape prevention programming on attitudes, behavior, and knowledge. *Journal of Counseling Psychology, 42,* 508-518.

Heppner, M. J., Neville, H. A., Smith, K., Kivlighan, D. M., & Gershuny, B. S. (1999). Examining immediate and long-term efficacy of rape prevention programming with racially diverse college men. *Journal of Counseling Psychology, 46,* 16-26.

Himelein, M. J. (1999). Acquaintance rape prevention with high-risk women: Identification and inoculation. *Journal of College Student Development, 40,* 93-96.

Holcomb, D. R., Sarvela, P. D., Sondag, K. A., & Holcomb, L. C. H. (1993). An evaluation of a mixed-gender date rape prevention workshop. *Journal of American College Health, 41,* 159-164.

Holtzworth-Munroe, A., Markman, H., O'Leary, K. D., Neidig, P., Leber, D., Heyman, R. E. et al. (1995). The need for marital violence prevention efforts: A behavioral-cognitive secondary prevention program for engaged and newly married couples. *Applied & Preventive Psychology, 4*, 77-88.

Holtzworth-Munroe, A., Waltz, J., Jacobson, N. S., Monaco, V., Fehrenbach, P. A., & Gottman, J. M. (1992). Recruiting non-violent couples as control subjects for research on marital violence: How easily can it be done? *Violence and Victims, 7*, 79-88.

Huesmann, L. R., Maxwell, C. D., Eron, L., Dahlberg, L. L., Guerra, N. G., Tolan, P. H. et al. (1996). Evaluating a cognitive/ecological program for the prevention of aggression among urban children. *American Journal of Preventive Medicine, 12*, 120-128.

Jaffe, P. G., Sudermann, M., Reitzel, D., & Killip, S. M. (1992). An evaluation of a secondary school primary prevention program on violence in intimate relationships. *Violence and Victims, 7*, 129-146.

Jones, L. E. (1991). The Minnesota School Curriculum Project: A statewide domestic violence prevention project in secondary schools. In B. Levy (Ed.), *Dating violence: Young women in danger* (pp. 258-266). Seattle, WA: Seal Press.

Koss, M. P., & Gidycz, C. A. (1985). Sexual experiences survey: Reliability and validity. *Journal of Consulting and Clinical Psychology, 53*, 422-423.

Krajewski, S. S., Rybarik, M. F., Dosch, M. E., & Gilmore, G. D. (1996). Results of a curriculum intervention with seventh graders regarding violence in relationships. *Journal of Family Violence, 11*, 93-112.

Kreft, I. G. G. (1997). The interactive effect of alcohol prevention programs in high school classes: An illustration of item homogeneity scaling and multilevel analysis techniques. In K. J. Bryant, M. Windle, & S. G. West (Eds.), *The science of prevention* (pp. 251-278). Washington, DC: American Psychological Association.

Laner, M. R. (1983). Courtship abuse and aggression: Contextual aspects. *Sociological Spectrum, 3*, 69-83.

Laner, M. R. (1989). Competition and combativeness in courtship: Reports from men. *Journal of Family Violence, 4*, 47-62.

Lanier, C. A., Elliott, M. N., Martin, D. W., & Kapadia, A. (1998). Evaluation of an intervention to change attitudes toward date rape. *Journal of American College Health, 46*, 177-180.

LaVant, B. (2001). Understanding violence on the college campuses and strategies for prevention. In D. S. Sandhu (Ed.), *Faces of violence: Psychological correlates, concepts, and intervention strategies* (pp. 45-71). Huntington, NY: Nova Science Publishers, Inc.

Lavoie, F., Vézina, L., Piché, C., & Boivin, M. (1995). Evaluation of a prevention program for violence in teen dating relationships. *Journal of Interpersonal Violence, 10*, 516-524.

Lenihan, G. O., Rawlins, M. E., Eberly, C. G., Buckley, B., & Masters, B. (1992). Gender differences in rape supportive attitudes before and after a date rape education intervention. *Journal of College Student Development, 33*, 331-338.

Levy, B. (1984). *Skills for violence-free relationships*. Santa Monica, CA: Southern California Coalition for Battered Women.

Linz, D., Fuson, I. A., & Donnerstein, E. (1990). Mitigating the negative effects of sexually violent mass communications through preexposure briefings. *Communication Research, 17*, 641-674.

Lipsey, M. W. (1992). Juvenile delinquency treatment: A meta-analytic inquiry into the variability of effects. In T. D. Cook, H. Cooper, D. S. Cordray, H. Hartman, L. V. Hedges, R. V. Light et al. (Eds.), *Meta-analysis for explanation* (pp. 83-127). Beverly Hills, CA: Sage.

Lipsey, M. W., & Wilson, D. B. (1993). The efficacy of psychological, educational, and behavioral treatment. *American Psychologist, 48*, 1181-1209.

Lonsway, K. A., Klaw, E. L., Berg, D. R., Waldo, C. R., Kothari, C., Mazurek, C. J. et al. (1998). Beyond "no means no": Outcomes of an intensive program to train peer facilitators for campus acquaintance rape education. *Journal of Interpersonal Violence, 13*, 73-92.

Lonsway, K. A., & Kothari, C. (2000). First year campus acquaintance rape education: Evaluating the impact of a mandatory intervention. *Psychology of Women Quarterly, 24*, 220-232.

Lorber, M. F., & O'Leary, K. D. (2004). Predictors of the persistence of male aggression in early marriage. *Journal of Family Violence, 19*, 329-333.

Lynam, D. R., Milich, R., Zimmerman, R., Novak, S. P., Logan, T. K., Martin, C. et al. (1999). Project DARE: No effects at 10-year follow-up. *Journal of Consulting and Clinical Psychology, 67*, 590-593.

Macgowan, M. J. (1997). An evaluation of a dating violence prevention program for middle school students. *Violence and Victims, 12*, 223-235.

Makepeace, J. M. (1981). Courtship violence among college students. *Family Relations, 30*, 97-102.

Malamuth, N. M. (1989). The attraction to sexual aggression scale: Part I. *Journal of Sex Research, 26*, 26-49.

Markman, H. J., Renick, M. J., Floyd, F. J., Stanley, S. M., & Clements, M. (1993). Preventing marital distress through communication and conflict management training: A 4- and 5-year follow-up. *Journal of Consulting and Clinical Psychology, 61*, 70-76.

Marlatt, G. A., Baer, J. S., Kivlahan, D. R., Dimeff, L. A., Larimer, M. E., Quigley, L. A. et al. (1998). Screening and brief intervention for high-risk college student drinkers: Results from a 2-year follow-up assessment. *Journal of Consulting and Clinical Psychology, 66*, 604-615.

Martin, S. E., & Bachman, R. (1997). The relationship of alcohol to injury in assault cases. In M. Galanter (Ed.), *Recent developments in alcoholism, Vol 13: Alcohol and violence: Epidemiology, neurobiology, psychology, family issues* (pp. 41-56). New York: Plenum Press.

Marx, B. P., Calhoun, K. S., Wilson, A. E., & Meyerson, L. A. (2001). Sexual revictimization prevention: An outcome evaluation. *Journal of Consulting and Clinical Psychology, 69*, 25-32.

Matthews, W. J. (1984). Violence in college couples. *College Student Journal, 8*, 150-158.

Miller, W. R. (1989). Increasing motivation for change. In R. K. Hester & W. R. Miller (Eds.), *Handbook of alcoholism treatment approaches: Effective alternatives* (pp. 67-79). Elmsford, NY: Pergamon Press.

Miller, W. R., Toscova, R. T., Miller, J. H., & Sanchez, V. (2000). A theory-based motivational approach for reducing alcohol/drug problems in college. *Health Education and Behavior, 27*, 744-759.

Moore, C. D., & Waterman, C. K. (1999). Predicting self-protection against sexual assault in dating relationships among heterosexual men and women, gay men, lesbians, and bisexuals. *Journal of College Student Development, 40*, 132-140.

Murray, D. M., Clark, M. H., & Wagenaar, A. C. (2000). Intraclass correlations from a community-based alcohol prevention study: The effect of repeat observations on the same communities. *Journal of Studies on Alcohol, 61*, 881-890.

Nelson, E. S., & Torgler, C. C. (1990). A comparison of strategies for changing college students' attitudes toward acquaintance rape. *Journal of Humanistic Education and Development, 29*, 69-85.

Office of Community Services, Administration for Children and Families. (1997). *Youth education and domestic violence model projects*. Laurel, MD: Laurel Consulting Group.

O'Keeffe, N. K., Brockopp, K., & Chew, E. (1986). Teen dating violence. *Social Work, 31*, 465-468.

O'Leary, K. D. (1999). Developmental and affective issues in assessing and treating partner aggression. *Clinical Psychology: Science and Practice, 6*, 400-414.

O'Leary, K.D., Barling, J., Arias, I., Rosenbaum, A., Malone, J., & Tyree, A. (1989). Prevalence and stability of marital aggression between spouses: A longitudinal analysis. *Journal of Consulting and Clinical Psychology, 57*, 263-268.

O'Leary, K. D., Vivian, D., & Malone, J. (1992). Assessment of physical aggression in marriage: The need for a multimodal assessment. *Behavioral Assessment, 14*, 5-14.

O'Leary, K. D., & Woodin, E. M. (2005). Bringing the agendas together: Partner and child abuse. In J. R. Lutzker (Ed.), *Violence prevention* (pp. 239-258). Washington, DC: American Psychological Association.

Orpinas, P., Kelder, S., Frankowski, R., Murray, N., Zhang, Q., & McAlister, A. (2000). Outcome evaluation of a multi-component violence-prevention program for middle schools: The Students for Peace project. *Health Education Research, 15*, 45-58.

Orpinas, P., Parcel, G. S., McAlister, A., & Frankowski, R. (1995). Violence prevention in middle schools: A pilot evaluation. *Journal of Adolescent Health, 17*, 360-371.

Pan, H. S., Neidig, P. H., & O'Leary, K. D. (1994). Predicting mild and severe husband-to-wife physical aggression. *Journal of Consulting and Clinical Psychology, 62*, 975-981.

Patton, W., & Mannison, M. (1993). Effects of a university subject on attitudes toward human sexuality. *Journal of Sex Education and Therapy, 19*, 93-107.

Perry, C. L., Williams, C. L., Veblen-Mortenson, S., Toomey, T., Komro, K., Anstine, P. S. et al. (1996). Outcomes of a community-wide alcohol use prevention program during early adolescence: Project Northland. *American Journal of Public Health, 86*, 956-965.

Pinzone-Glover, H. A., Gidycz, C. A., & Jacobs, C. D. (1998). An acquaintance rape prevention program: Effects on attitudes toward women, rape-related attitudes, and perceptions of rape scenarios. *Psychology of Women Quarterly, 22*, 605-621.

Pittman, A. L., Wolfe, D. A., & Wekerle, C. (2000). Strategies for evaluating dating violence prevention programs. *Journal of Aggression, Maltreatment & Trauma, 4*, 217-238.

Quigley, B. M., & Leonard, K. E. (1996). Desistance from marital violence in the early years of marriage. *Violence and Victims, 11,* 355-370.

Robinson, W. S. (1950). Ecological correlations and the behavior of individuals. *Sociological Review, 15,* 351-357.

Roscoe, B., & Callahan, J. E. (1985). Adolescents' self-report of violence in families and dating relations. *Adolescence, 20,* 545-553.

Rosenthal, E. H., Heesacker, M., & Neimeyer, G. J. (1995). Changing the rape-supportive attitudes of traditional and nontraditional male and female college students. *Journal of Counseling Psychology, 42,* 171-177.

Schaeffer, A. M., & Nelson, E. S. (1993). Rape-supportive attitudes: Effects of on-campus residence and education. *Journal of College Student Development, 34,* 175-179.

Schewe, P. A., & O'Donohue, W. (1993). Sexual abuse prevention with high-risk males: The roles of victim empathy and rape myths. *Violence and Victims, 8,* 339-351.

Schewe, P. A., & O'Donohue, W. (1996). Rape prevention with high-risk males: Short-term outcome of two interventions. *Archives of Sexual Behavior, 25,* 455-471.

Schumacher, J. A., Feldbau-Kohn, S., Slep, A. M. S., & Heyman, R. E. (2001). Risk factors for male-to-female partner physical abuse. *Aggression & Violent Behavior, 6,* 281-352.

Straus, M. A. (1979). Measuring intrafamily conflict and violence: The conflict tactics (CT) scales. *Journal of Marriage and the Family, 41,* 75-86.

Straus, M. A., & Gelles, R. J. (Eds.). (1990). *Physical violence in American families.* New Brunswick, NJ: Transaction.

Sussman, S., Lichtman, K., Ritt, A., & Pallonen, U.E. (1999). Effects of thirty-four adolescent tobacco use cessation and prevention trials on regular users of tobacco products. *Substance Use and Misuse, 34,* 1469-1503.

Tobler, N. S., & Stratton, H. H. (1997). Effectiveness of school-based drug prevention programs: A meta-analysis of the research. *Journal of Primary Prevention, 18,* 71-128.

Walter, H. J. (2001). School-based prevention of problem behaviors. *School Consultation/Intervention, 10,* 117-127.

Walters, S. T., & Bennett, M. E. (2000). Addressing drinking among college students: A review of the empirical literature. *Alcoholism Treatment Quarterly, 18,* 61-77.

Walters, S. T., Bennett, M. E., & Noto, J. V. (2000). Drinking on campus: What do we know about reducing alcohol use among college students? *Journal of Substance Abuse Treatment, 19,* 223-228.

Weisz, A. N., & Black, B. M. (2001). Evaluating a sexual assault and dating violence prevention program for urban youths. *Social Work Research, 25,* 89-102.

Wekerle, C., & Wolfe, D. A. (1998). Prevention of physical abuse and neglect: Windows of opportunity. In P. K. Trickett & C. Schellenbach (Eds.), *Violence against children in the family and the community* (pp. 339-370). New York: APA Books.

Wekerle, C., & Wolfe, D. A. (1999). Dating violence in mid-adolescence: Theory, significance, and emerging prevention initiatives. *Clinical Psychology Review, 19,* 435-456.

Widom, C. S. (1989). Does violence beget violence? A critical examination of the literature. *Psychological Bulletin, 106,* 3-28.

Williams, C. L., & Perry, C. L. (1998). Lessons from Project Northland: Preventing alcohol problems during adolescence. *Alcohol Health and Research World, 22,* 107-116.

Wilson, D. B., Gottfredson, D. C., & Najaka, S. S. (2001). School-based prevention of problem behaviors: A meta-analysis. *Journal of Quantitative Criminology, 17,* 247-272.

Wilson, J. Q., & Herrnstein, R. J. (1985). *Crime and human nature.* New York: Simon & Schuster.

Wolfe, D. A., Wekerle, C., Scott, K., Straatman, A., Grasley, C., & Reitzel-Jaffe, D. (2003). Dating violence prevention with at-risk youth: A controlled outcome evaluation. *Journal of Consulting and Clinical Psychology, 71,* 279-291.

Wolfe, D. A., Wekerle, C., Gough, R., Reitzel-Jaffe, D., Grasley, C., Pittman, A. et al. (1996). *Youth Relationships Manual: A group approach with adolescents for the prevention of woman abuse and the promotion of healthy relationships.* Thousand Oaks, CA: Sage.

Wynn, S. R., Schulenberg, J., Maggs, J. L., & Zucker, R. A. (2000). Preventing alcohol misuse: The impact of refusal skills and norms. *Psychology of Addictive Behaviors, 14,* 36-47.

Yllo, K. (1993). Through a feminist lens: Gender, power, and violence. In R. J. Gelles & D. R. Loseke (Eds.), *Current controversies in family violence* (pp. 47-62). Newbury Park, CA: Sage.

Yung, B. R., & Hammond, W. R. (1998). Breaking the cycle: A culturally sensitive violence prevention program for African-American children and adolescents. In J. R. Lutzker (Ed.), *Handbook of child abuse research and treatment* (pp. 319-340). New York: Plenum Press.

doi:10.1300/J146v13n03_06

APPENDIX. Dating Violence Prevention Programs

Program Description	Method	Target(s) for Change
Dating Aggression Programs		
Avery-Leaf et al., 1997. Didactic, skill-based, universal dating violence prevention program. Five-session curriculum for high school health classes. <u>Facilitators</u>: Health teachers attend 8-hour training seminar one week prior to program implementation.	<u>Design</u>: Two-condition pretest-posttest quasi-experimental design. <u>Participants</u>: 193 white (79.8%), lower-middle class students (106 males & 87 females) enrolled in health classes (grades 11-12) at a suburban US high school. <u>Objectives</u>: Promote equity in dating relationships, effective communication, help seeking, conflict resolution, and challenge attitudes toward violence.	Attitudinal justification of violence (self-report).
Jaffe et al., 1992. Universal dating violence prevention program targeting students, administrators, teachers, & parents. Single-session curriculum consisting of either 1/2 day (90-minute auditorium presentation & 60-minute classroom discussion) or full-day (1/2-day curriculum plus development of action plans) intervention implemented in high schools. <u>Facilitators</u>: Service providers who lead discussions attend half-day training seminar and follow-up at 6-weeks.	<u>Design</u>: One-group (intervention only) pretest, posttest, (6-week) follow-up design; stratified sampling by grade and program from 4 schools. <u>Participants</u>: 737 predominantly white students (379 males & 358 females) in grades 9 to 13 from 4 Canadian high schools. <u>Objectives</u>: Define abuse, address myths regarding wife abuse, challenge attitudes about violence against women and promote help-seeking behaviors.	Attitudes, knowledge, and behavioral intentions regarding relationship violence (self-report questionnaire designed for study).
Lavoie et al., 1995. Didactic, universal program of dating violence prevention. Short-Form Curriculum: Two classroom sessions (120-150 minutes total); Long-Form Curriculum: Short-Form + viewing a dating violence film & writing fictional letters (to a victim and to a perpetrator; additional 120-150 minutes) for flexible implementation in any high school classroom. <u>Facilitators</u>: Community service provider and volunteer trained by project staff.	<u>Design</u>: Two-condition intervention (short- or long-form), pretest-posttest design. <u>Participants</u>: 517 10th-grade students (222 males & 295 females; 279 short-form & 238 long-form) from 2 Canadian high schools. Demographics unclear. <u>Objectives</u>: Identify and distinguish between different forms of control, increase knowledge about partner violence, and promote equity in dating relationships.	Attitudes and knowledge about dating violence (self-report questionnaire designed for study).

APPENDIX (continued)

Program Description	Method	Target(s) for Change
	Dating Aggression Programs	
Macgowan, 1997. Didactic, skills-based, universal dating violence prevention program. Five-session curriculum (each session 60 minutes) for flexible implementation in schools. <u>Facilitators</u>: Teachers attend a 3-hour training session lead by project staff.	<u>Design</u>: Pretest-posttest wait-list control group, quasi-experimental design. Stratified sampling by grade (6-8) and level (regular or advanced). <u>Participants</u>: 440 (193 males & 247 females) predominantly Black, non-Hispanic (72.3%) students from a junior high school in an American city. <u>Objectives</u>: Increase knowledge about dating violence, and promote equity in dating relationships, effective communication, and help seeking.	Attitudes and knowledge about dating violence.
Minnesota School Curriculum Project (Jones, 1991). Didactic, skill-based, universal & secondary DV prevention program with dating violence section added for senior high students. Number of sessions not specified. <u>Facilitators</u>: Teachers trained by project staff and community service members.	<u>Design</u>: Two-group pretest-posttest quasi-experimental. <u>Participants</u>: 560 junior high & 600 high school students in Minnesota almost equally divided between experimental and control groups. Demographics not specified. <u>Objectives</u>: Define abuse, address myths regarding wife abuse, and increase knowledge about partner violence and community services.	Attitudes and knowledge about domestic violence.
Prevention and Relationship Enhancement Program (PREP; Markman et al., 1993). Didactic, skills-based universal prevention program utilizing cognitive-behavioral and communication-oriented marital therapy techniques. Five-session curriculum program (each session 180 minutes). <u>Facilitators</u>: Advanced undergraduate psychology students or graduate clinical psychology students attend a 20-hour training.	<u>Design</u>: Two-condition, multiple assessment (pretest, 8- to 10-week posttest, and 1.5-, 3-, 4- and 5-year follow-up) design. <u>Participants</u>: 75 community couples (25 intervention, 50 controls) planning marriage selected from a larger sample. <u>Objectives</u>: Promote effective communication and conflict management skills, maintain high levels of relationship functioning, and prevent future relationship problems.	Relationship functioning, relationship satisfaction, communication and conflict-management skills, and the frequency of physical violence.

Program Description	Method	Target(s) for Change
	Dating Aggression Programs	
The Safe Dates Project (Foshee et al., 1996). Universal and secondary prevention program of dating violence among youth. Process-oriented, semi-structured discussion (ten 45-minute sessions) and activity based (role-playing, student plays, poster contest) intervention. <u>Facilitators</u>: Health teachers attend a 20-hour training seminar lead by staff members.	<u>Design</u>: Two-condition experimental design (at the school level). Pretest-posttest, one-month and one-year follow-ups. Stratified sampling by grade from 14 schools (7 treatment and 7 control) random assignment to condition. <u>Participants</u>: 1965 Caucasian (79.5%) 8th & 9th grade students (975 males and 990 females) from a rural area. <u>Objectives</u>: Increase knowledge about dating violence, challenge attitudes toward violence and gender stereotyping, and promote equity in dating relationships, effective communication, conflict resolution, and help-seeking.	Attitudes about dating violence, conflict resolution skills, and help-seeking behaviors (based on self-report).
Skills for Violence-Free Relationships (Levy, 1984; Krajewski et al., 1996). Didactic, skills-based universal prevention program for woman abuse. Ten-session curriculum implemented in health class. <u>Facilitators</u>: The health teacher and the counselor from a local battered women's shelter attended a day-long training session lead by the director of the shelter.	<u>Design</u>: Quasi-experimental nonequivalent control group design. Pretest, posttest, and five-month follow-up. <u>Participants</u>: 239 primarily Caucasian (78.8%) seventh grade students from two Midwestern junior high schools. <u>Objectives</u>: Increase knowledge about woman abuse, challenge attitudes toward violence, challenge sex role stereotypes, and promote effective conflict resolution.	Attitudes and knowledge about partner abuse.
Youth Relationship Project (Wolfe et al., 1996, 2003). Process-oriented, semi-structured, interactive, skill-based, targeted prevention program for dating violence. 18-session curriculum (each session 120 minutes) currently implemented as a weekly after school program. <u>Facilitators</u>: Community service providers who attend a two-day (10-hour) training seminar. All sessions led by one females and one male facilitator.	<u>Design</u>: Two-condition multi-method, multi-respondent, multiple assessment (pre-, mid-, & post-group and a detailed follow-up schedule) experimental design. <u>Participants</u>: 191 Caucasian (85%) child protective custody youth (92 males and 99 females) with a history of childhood maltreatment. <u>Objectives</u>: Increase knowledge about dating violence and promote conflict resolution, effective communication, help-seeking and social action.	Attitudes and knowledge about partner abuse, violence behavior in dating relationships, communication and conflict resolution skills, and help-seeking and social action skills.

APPENDIX (continued)

Program Description	Method	Target(s) for Change
Dating Aggression Programs		
Combined Dating and Sexual Aggression Programs		
Weisz & Black, 2001. Universal, 12-session (90 minutes each) program of dating and sexual violence among youth. Process-oriented, semi-structured discussion and activity based (role-playing, modeling, experiential exercises) intervention. Facilitators: Two male and two female co-trainers who possessed MSW degrees or were enrolled in MSW programs.	Design: Two-condition, quasi-experimental pretest-posttest-follow-up design. Participants: 66 African-American intercity youth in seventh grade. Objectives: Increasing knowledge about and intolerance for dating and sexual aggression and promoting behaviors inconsistent with sexual assault and dating violence.	Knowledge, attitudes, and behaviors related to sexual assault and dating aggression.
Sexual Assault Programs		
Acquaintance Rape Prevention Program (Gray et al., 1990). Universal, didactic, skill-based program for women.	Design: Two-condition (personalized vs. standard intervention), pretest-posttest experimental design (random assignment at the class level). Participants: 70 predominantly Caucasian (74%) women attending a community college in a rural area. Objectives: Reduce risk-taking behaviors.	Intent to engage in risky behavior and perception of vulnerability to acquaintance rape.
Anderson et al., 1998. Universal, one-session (60 minute) interventions consisting of either a video or an interactive mock talk show. Facilitators: Counseling psychology graduate students who received 6 months of training at the university counseling center (a licensed psychologist also participated in the mock talk show).	Design: Three-condition (video, talk show, no-treatment control), pretest-posttest-follow-up design. Participants: 215 (143 females, 72 males) predominantly Caucasian (90%) undergraduate students attending a Midwestern university. Objectives: Decrease rape myth acceptance and attitudes tolerant of rape.	Rape myth acceptance and attitudes toward rape.
Black et al., 2000. Universal, theatrical performance about sexual aggression followed by group discussions about the performance and topics related to sexual assault. Facilitators: Peer educators who completed 40-hours of training and who worked with a theater consultant approximately 17 hours over an 8-week period.	Design: Two condition, quasi-experimental pretest-posttest-follow-up design. Participants: 164 (124 females, 40 males) students and residents of the Metro-Detroit area. Objectives: Decrease rape myth acceptance.	Attitudes toward sexual assault.

Program Description	Method	Target(s) for Change
	Sexual Assault Programs	
Berg et al., 1999. Universal, one-session (75 minutes) empathy induction program. Facilitators: Two trained male presenters.	Design: Three-condition (listen to an audiotape of a female rape victim, a male rape victim or a didactic presentation about rape), pretest-posttest quasi-experimental design. Participants: 54 predominantly Caucasian (74%) college males attending a Midwestern university. Objectives: Reduce rape-supportive attitudes and likelihood to engage in rape-supportive behaviors and induce empathy for rape victims.	Likelihood of engaging in sexually aggressive behaviors, rape myth acceptance, rape-supportive attitudes, and general empathy and empathy specific to rape.
Breitenbecher & Gidycz, 1998. Didactic, process-oriented program targeted toward women with a history of sexual victimization.	Design: Two-condition quasi-experimental, pretest-posttest design. Participants: 406 primarily Caucasian (95%) women attending a Midwestern university. Objectives: Increase awareness of the pervasiveness of and association between sexual assault and revictimization, decrease rape myth acceptance, and encourage behaviors inconsistent with sexual assault (re)victimization.	Likelihood of sexual revictimization, risky dating behaviors, sexual communication, and sexual assault awareness.
Breitenbecher & Scarce, 1999. Universal, one-session (60-minute) didactic program for females. Facilitator: Graduate student who received extensive training.	Design: Two-condition experimental design; Pretest and seven-month follow-up; Participants: 224 primarily Caucasian women attending a Midwestern university. Objectives: Increase knowledge about rape, challenge sex role stereotypes, and decrease risk for sexual victimization.	Attitudes and knowledge about sexual assault and behaviors associated with risk of sexual victimization.
Breitenbecher & Scarce, 2001. Universal, one-session (90-minute) didactic, skills-based program for females.	Design: Two-condition experimental design; Pretest and seven-month follow-up. Participants: 94 primarily Caucasian undergraduate women attending a Midwestern university. Objectives: Increase knowledge about rape, challenge sex role stereotypes, and decrease risk for sexual victimization.	Attitudes and knowledge about sexual assault and behaviors associated with risk of sexual victimization.

APPENDIX (continued)

Program Description	Method	Target(s) for Change
Sexual Assault Programs		
Campus Acquaintance Rape Education (CARE) (Lonsway et al., 1998). Universal, semester-long, comprehensive university course that trains undergraduate students to facilitate campus peer workshops. Facilitator: CARE program coordinator with undergraduate and graduate assistants.	Design: Two-condition (human sexuality course vs. CARE program) quasi-experimental pretest-posttest-follow-up design. Participants: 170 (111 females, 59 males) undergraduate students enrolled either in CARE or human sexuality courses at a Midwestern university. Objectives: Reduce rape myth acceptance and endorsement of adversarial sexual beliefs and increase support for feminist movement and assertive responses to sexual conflict scenarios.	Rape myth acceptance, adversarial sexual beliefs, and attitudes toward women.
Dallager & Rosén, 1993. Universal, Human Sexuality course. Facilitators: Instructor with a feministic orientation.	Design: Two-condition, pretest-posttest quasi-experimental design. Participants: 145 (47 males, 98 females) predominantly Caucasian (90%) undergraduate students enrolled in Human Sexuality and Education courses at a Midwestern university. Objectives: Decrease rape myth and interpersonal aggression acceptance.	Rape myth and interpersonal aggression acceptance.
Earle, 1996. Universal didactic sexual assault programs at three Northeastern colleges.	Design: Four condition (3 colleges' sexual assault programs and 1 one college with no sexual assault program), pretest-posttest, quasi-experimental design. Participants: 347 first-year college men attending four Northeastern colleges. Objectives: Challenge rape-accepting attitudes and attitudes about traditional gender roles.	Attitudes toward rape and women.
Ellis et al., 1992. Universal, one-session intervention consisting of imaginal exposure.	Design: Pretest-posttest design. Participants: 151 (100 females, 51 males) undergraduates. Objectives: Decreased endorsement of rape supportive attitudes and myths.	Attitudes toward rape and rape mythology.

Program Description	Method	Target(s) for Change
	Sexual Assault Programs	
Feltey et al., 1991. Universal, one-session (45 minutes) didactic program. Facilitator: YWCA rape educator.	Design: Pretest-posttest design. Participants: 118 (41 males, 77 females) predominantly Caucasian (71%) high school students. Objectives: Challenge sexual coercion attitudes.	Sexual coercion attitudes.
First Year Campus Acquaintance Rape Education (FYCARE) (Lonsway & Kothari, 2000). Universal, one-session (120 minute) didactic program. Facilitators: Graduate and undergraduate peer educators who completed a semester-long training course.	Design: Three-condition (FYCARE participants assessed immediately after program, FYCARE participants sampled through the unrelated context of introductory psychology courses, and a no-treatment control), quasi-experimental design. Participants: 191 (89 females, 102 males) predominantly Caucasian (73%) undergraduate students attending a Midwestern university. Objectives: Heighten awareness of rape and relevant campus services, challenge rape myths and rape-acceptant attitudes, and increase personal responsibility to stop rape in own and others' lives.	Rape myth acceptance and attitudes and knowledge about rape.
Fonow et al., 1992. Universal, one-session didactic curriculum.	Design: Three-condition (video, workshop, or no-treatment control) experimental design (random assignment at the class section level). Pretest-posttest and posttest only designs. Participants: 582 (319 females; 263 males) predominantly Caucasian (86%) students attending a Midwestern university. Objectives: Increase knowledge about rape and reduce rape-myth acceptance.	Knowledge and attitudes about rape.
Frazier et al., 1994. Universal, interactive improvisational theater performance. Facilitators: Counselors from the campus sexual violence program.	Design: Two-condition, pretest-posttest-follow-up quasi-experimental design. Participants: 192 (75 males, 117 females) predominantly Caucasian (97%) students in fraternities or sororities at a Midwestern university. Objectives: Decrease attitudes and behaviors that foster acquaintance rape and encouraging equality and respect between men and women, assertive communication, and safety precautions for women.	Attitudes towards dating and sexual behaviors and gender role beliefs.

APPENDIX (continued)

Program Description	Method	Target(s) for Change
Sexual Assault Programs		
Gidycz, Layman et al., 2001. Universal, one-session didactic curriculum.	Design: Two-condition, pretest-posttest design. Participants: 1,108 (300 males, 808 females) primarily Caucasian (93%) undergraduates attending a Midwestern university. Objectives: Increase knowledge about rape, reduce rape-myth acceptance and risk of sexual assault, and increase personal safety and help-seeking behaviors.	Attitudes toward women, rape, and rape mythology, level of rape empathy, and sexual assault perpetration (for males) and victimization (for females).
Gilbert et al., 1991. Universal one-session (60-minute) didactic program for men.	Design: Two-condition, pretest-posttest-follow-up experimental design. Participants: 61 predominantly Caucasian (87%) undergraduate men from two U.S. universities. Objectives: Challenge attitudes toward dating and sexual violence and gender stereotyping.	Attitudes about dating and sexual aggression, motivation, and understandability and subjective evaluation of the program.
Hanson & Gidycz, 1993. Universal, didactic program for women. Facilitator: First author.	Design: Two-condition, pretest-posttest experimental design. Participants: 346 predominantly Caucasian (94%) undergraduate women from a large U.S. university. Objectives: Increase sexual assault awareness, dispel common rape myths, foster effective sexual communication, reduce incidence of sexual assault and risky dating behaviors.	Likelihood of sexual victimization, risky dating behaviors, sexual communication, and sexual assault awareness.
Harrison et al., 1991. Universal, one-session interventions consisting of either a videotaped presentation or the video plus a group discussion.	Design: Three-condition (video treatment group, video plus facilitated discussion treatment group, and a no-treatment control) pretest-posttest experimental design. Participants: 96 students from a large southwestern public university. Objectives: Decreased endorsement of rape supportive attitudes and myths.	Attitudes about rape.

Program Description	Method	Target(s) for Change
	Sexual Assault Programs	
Heppner, Good et al., 1995. Universal one-session (60 minutes) didactic program. Facilitator: An expert in rape prevention programming.	Design: Pretest-posttest-follow-up design. Participants: 257 (152 females, 105 males) predominantly Caucasian (89%) undergraduate students attending a Midwestern university. Objectives: Decrease adversarial sexual beliefs and rape myth acceptance.	Adversarial sexual beliefs, rape myth acceptance, central route change mechanisms.
Heppner, Humphrey et al., 1995. Universal, one-session (90 minutes) didactic-video program and innovative, interactive drama performance. Facilitators: One male and one female counseling psychology doctoral students with two years experience with rape education.	Design: Three-condition (didactic-video program; innovative, interactive drama; no-treatment control), pretest-posttest-multiple follow-up, experimental design. Participants: 258 (129 males, 129 females) predominantly Caucasian (93%) undergraduate students attending a Midwestern university. Objectives: Decrease rape myth acceptance, increase ability to discriminate coercion from consent and willingness to volunteer time to help in rape prevention activities and to support a fee increase for rape prevention, and promote thought and discussion about the intervention.	Rape myth acceptance, central route change mechanisms, ability to discriminate coercion from consent, willingness to volunteer time to help in rape prevention and to support a fee increase, and amount of thought and discussion generated by interventions.
Heppner et al., 1999. Universal, three-session (90-minutes each) didactic and skills-based curriculum for men (one standard and one culturally relevant). Facilitators: Three male facilitators who received approximately 25 hours of training (one facilitator was a staff member of the campus Rape Education office).	Design: Three-condition (culturally relevant treatment, regular treatment, and no-treatment control) pretest-posttest-follow-up design. Participants: 119 predominantly Caucasian (64%) undergraduate males at a large Midwestern university (most were in two campus fraternities). Objectives: Reduce rape supportive attitudes, facilitate understanding of the emotional needs of rape victims, and provide repertoires for helping victims.	Attitudes toward rape, and rape mythology, likelihood for central route attitude change to occur, sexual assault behavioral intent, and sexual assault perpetration (for males).

APPENDIX (continued)

Program Description	Method	Target(s) for Change
	Sexual Assault Program	
Holcomb et al., 1993. Universal, one-session (35-minute) intervention. Facilitators: Male and female cofacilitators.	Design: Two-condition, posttest-only experimental design (at the class level). (Modified and randomized control-group.) Participants: 331 (173 males and 158) predominantly Caucasian (87%) students from a large Midwestern university. Objectives: Decreased endorsement of rape supportive attitudes.	Attitudes toward rape.
Himelein, 1999. Didactic, process-oriented five-session curriculum (90 minutes each) targeted for women at high risk for sexual assault. Facilitators: Author (licensed clinical psychologist) and two senior psychology majors who completed approximately 40 hours of training.	Design: Pretest-posttest design. Participants: 7 women at high risk for sexual assault. Objectives: Increase knowledge about sexual assault and decrease risky dating behaviors.	Knowledge about sexual assault and risky dating behaviors.
How to Help a Sexual Assault Survivor (Foubert & Marriott, 1997). Universal one-session didactic curriculum for males. Facilitators: Male undergraduate peer educators.	Design: Two-condition, pretest-posttest-follow-up quasi-experimental design. Participants: 109 predominantly Caucasian (97%) fraternity members. Objectives: Decrease rape myth acceptance and likelihood of sexual assault perpetration.	Rape myth acceptance and likelihood of sexual assault perpetration.
How to Help a Sexual Assault Survivor: What Men Can Do (Foubert & McEwen, 1998). Universal, one-session (60 minutes) didactic program for men. Facilitators: Four male peer educators.	Design: Two-condition, quasi-experimental pretest-posttest and pretest-only designs. Participants: 155 predominantly Caucasian (88%) members from six fraternities at a large mid-Atlantic university Objectives: Decreased rape myth acceptance and behavioral intent to rape.	Rape myth acceptance, behavioral intent to rape, and central route change mechanisms.

Program Description	Method	Target(s) for Change
Sexual Assault Program		
Lanier et al., 1998. Universal, six-scene play depicting various sexual assault situations.	Design: Two-condition, pretest-posttest quasi-experimental design. Participants: 436 predominantly Caucasian (65%) undergraduates from a private southern university. Objectives: Combat rape-tolerant attitudes and decrease risk for sexual perpetration and victimization.	Attitudes about sexual assault and behaviors associated with risk of sexual perpetration and victimization.
Lenihan et al., 1992. Universal, one-session (50-minute) didactic program. Facilitators: Two sexual assault crisis counselors and two residence hall counselors.	Design: Solomon four-group design. Participants: 821 (503 females and 318 males) undergraduate students attending a Midwestern university. Objectives: Challenge rape-accepting attitudes.	Attitudes toward rape and rape mythology.
Linz et al., 1990. Universal, one-session didactic program.	Design: Five condition (three experimental, two control: videotaped reading essay about sexual violence + watching the tape, videotaped reading essay about sexual violence + no playback, essay about media use + playback, neutral information presented, no information), pretest-posttest experimental design. Participants: 44 undergraduate males enrolled in an introductory communication course. Objectives: Decrease acceptance of rape myths and interpersonal violence and perpetration of sexually coercive behaviors.	Rape myth acceptance, attitudes about interpersonal aggression, sexually coercive behaviors, and perceived responsibility of rape perpetrators and victims.
Marx et al., 2001. Two-session (60-minutes each) didactic, skills-based program targeted for women with a history of sexual victimization. Facilitators: Trained, master's-level female graduate-research assistants.	Design: Two-condition, pretest-posttest experimental design. Participants: 61 predominantly Caucasian (85%) undergraduate women with a history of sexual victimization from two U.S. universities. Objectives: Reduce sexual revictimization, increasing knowledge about sexual assault, provide strategies for decreasing risk of sexual assault, and fostering effective problem-solving, assertiveness, and communication skills.	Likelihood of revictimization, psychopathology, self-efficacy ratings of several behaviors specific to sexual situations, and risk recognition.

APPENDIX (continued)

Program Description	Method	Target(s) for Change
	Sexual Assault Program	
Moore & Waterman, 1999. Exposure to rape-prevention education (e.g., through books or articles on sexual assault, college courses in which rape prevention was discussed).	Design: Correlational. Participants: 152 (63 males, 87 females, 2 unreported) predominantly Caucasian (74%) college students recruited from various classes or campus organizations. Objectives: Investigate whether exposure to rape-prevention education is positively related to self-protecting dating behaviors.	Self-protective dating behaviors.
Nelson & Torgler, 1990. Universal, one-session (either 10 or 30 minutes) didactic programs (brochure or video).	Design: Three-condition (video, written material, control) pretest-posttest quasi-experimental design. Participants: 89 (25 males; 64 females) undergraduate students Objectives: Reduce rape-accepting attitudes and promote less traditional attitudes toward women.	Attitudes toward women and rape.
Ohio University Sexual Assault Risk Reduction Program (Gidycz, Lynn et al., 2001). Universal one-session (180-minute) didactic program with interactive components. Facilitators: Trained graduate students.	Design: Two-condition, pretest-posttest-follow-up experimental design. Participants: 762 predominantly Caucasian undergraduate women from two U. S. universities. Objectives: Increase awareness of sexual assault risk, assertive defensive behaviors, and help seeking behaviors and reduce victim blaming and (re)victimization.	Likelihood of (re)victimization, risky dating behaviors, sexual communication, and rape empathy.
Patton & Mannison, 1993. Universal, Human Sexuality course.	Design: Three-condition (undergraduate human sexuality course; graduate human sexuality course; control), pretest-posttest quasi-experimental design. Participants: 115 (25 males, 90 females) students enrolled in Human Sexuality or Education courses at Queensland University of Technology in Australia. Objectives: Increased awareness of sexuality issues.	Attitudes towards sexuality.

Program Description	Method	Target(s) for Change
Sexual Assault Program		
Pinzone-Glover et al., 1998. Universal, one-session (60 minutes) didactic program. Facilitators: Two male and two female psychology graduate students.	Design: Two-condition (sexually transmitted disease presentation, rape-prevention program) Participants: 152 (93 females, 59 males) predominantly Caucasian (85%) undergraduate students attending two Midwestern universities. Objectives: Reduce rape myth acceptance, and increase empathy toward rape victims, positive attitudes toward women, and the ability to identify and define rape situations.	Rape myth acceptance, empathy towards rape victims or perpetrators, attitudes toward women, and ability to identify rape situations.
Rosenthal et al., 1995. Universal, one-session (60 minutes) didactic program. Facilitators: One man with a counseling degree and one undergraduate woman.	Design: Two-condition, pretest-posttest-follow-up experimental design. Participants: 245 (123 female, 122 male) predominantly white undergraduate students attending a southern university who tended to score either high or low on Burt's (1980) Sex Role Stereotyping. Objectives: Reduce rape myth acceptance and rape-supportive attitudes.	Rape myth acceptance and rape-supportive attitudes.
Schaeffer & Nelson, 1993. Universal classes or programs about sexual violence.	Design: Posttest-only design. Participants: 160 male undergraduate students attending a southeastern university living in one of the following conditions: single-sex residence halls, co-ed residence halls, and fraternity houses. Objectives: Decrease rape myth acceptance and promote less traditional beliefs in gender roles.	Rape myth acceptance and beliefs about gender roles.
Schewe & O'Donohue, 1993. Didactic, 45-minute video presentations targeted at men at risk for perpetration of sexual aggression. Facilitators: Trained graduate students.	Design: Three-condition (empathy treatment, facts treatment, no-treatment control), pretest-posttest, quasi-experimental design. Participants: 55 (42 high-risk, 13 low-risk) male undergraduate students attending a Midwestern university. Objectives: Increase empathy toward sexual abuse victims, and decrease attitudes accepting of interpersonal aggression and rape, the likelihood of perpetration of sexual abuse, sexual harassment, and rape, and arousal to rape.	Empathy toward sexual abuse victims, likelihood of perpetrating sexual abuse, sexual harassment, and rape, attitudes and adversarial beliefs about interpersonal violence and rape, and arousal to rape.

APPENDIX (continued)

Program Description	Method	Target(s) for Change
Sexual Assault Program		
Schewe & O'Donohue, 1996. Victim Empathy/Outcome Expectancies Intervention (VE/OE) and Rape Supportive Cognitions Intervention (RSC)–Didactic, one-session programs targeted at men who score high on a measure of attraction to sexual aggression (both included videotaped presentations and an interactive exercise; VE/OE also included a group discussion).	<u>Design</u>: Three-condition (RSC, VE/OE Intervention, No-treatment control) quasi-experimental design. <u>Participants</u>: 74 predominantly Caucasian undergraduate men from a Midwestern university who scored above a score of 14 on the Attraction to Sexual Aggression scale (Malamuth, 1989). <u>Objectives</u>: Of VE/OE–change outcome expectancies of rape; Of RSC–Increase knowledge about sexual communication, rape myths, and consequences of rape.	Attitudes and knowledge about the consequences of rape, sexual communication, and rape myths.
The Men's Program (Foubert, 2000). Universal, one-session (60-minute) didactic program for males. <u>Facilitators</u>: Four male peer educators.	<u>Design</u>: Two-condition experimental design (at the fraternity level; eight fraternities total). Combination of pretest-posttest/follow-up and posttest-only designs. <u>Participants</u>: 147 predominantly Caucasian (91%) undergraduate fraternity members from a mid-Atlantic university. <u>Objectives</u>: Decrease acceptance of rape myths, behavioral intent to rape, and sexually coercive behavior.	Attitudes about rape, behavioral intent to rape, and sexually coercive behavior.

This Appendix was adopted from Pittman, Wolfe, and Wekerle's (2000) Table 1. Given that a number of reviews of sexual assault prevention programs have been published, we only reviewed programs published from 1990 to the present.

The Who, What, When, Where, and How of Partner Violence Prevention Research

Sherry L. Hamby

SUMMARY. Fundamental questions remain unanswered about partner violence prevention programs. These include issues of the appropriate scope, format, audience, setting, and mechanics of partner violence prevention. Should partner violence prevention be included in general curricula that address several problem behaviors or be taught in specialized programs? Should partner violence prevention be universally directed towards all youth, all adults, targeted to high-risk subgroups, or some combination? Should partner violence prevention instruction focus more on protective or risk factors? How do factors such as attendance, program integrity, and facilitator skill affect outcome? Existing information on these issues is considered, including data from related fields. Studies comparing different types of programs, including cost-benefit studies, are urgently needed in order to make informed program and policy decisions. doi:10.1300/J146v13n03_07 *[Article copies available for a fee from The Haworth Document Delivery Service: 1-800-HAWORTH. E-mail address: <docdelivery@haworthpress.com> Website: <http://www.HaworthPress.com> © 2006 by The Haworth Press, Inc. All rights reserved.]*

Address correspondence to: Sherry L. Hamby, PhD, Possible Equalities, P.O. Box 772, Laurinburg, NC 28353 (E-mail: slhamby@email.unc.edu).

The author would like to thank Becky Buehler for suggestions on an earlier draft of this paper.

Presented May 14, 2002, at the Department of Defense Maltreatment Prevention Symposium, Arlington, VA.

[Haworth co-indexing entry note]: "The Who, What, When, Where, and How of Partner Violence Prevention Research." Hamby, Sherry L. Co-published simultaneously in *Journal of Aggression, Maltreatment & Trauma* (The Haworth Maltreatment & Trauma Press, an imprint of The Haworth Press, Inc.) Vol. 13, No. 3/4, 2006, pp. 179-201; and: *Prevention of Intimate Partner Violence* (ed: Sandra M. Stith) The Haworth Maltreatment & Trauma Press, an imprint of The Haworth Press, Inc., 2006, pp. 179-201. Single or multiple copies of this article are available for a fee from The Haworth Document Delivery Service [1-800-HAWORTH, 9:00 a.m. - 5:00 p.m. (EST). E-mail address: docdelivery@haworthpress.com].

KEYWORDS. Prevention, partner violence, program evaluation, cost-benefit analyses, policy

It may seem surprising today, but it was not until 1986 when the first formal evaluation of a partner violence prevention program appeared (Walther, 1986). It would be the 1990s before more followed it (Jaffe, Suderman, Reitzel, & Killip, 1992; Jones, 1991). This despite the fact that the modern social movement against partner violence began in the early 1970s, and from the beginning included efforts to intervene with families already experiencing violence (e.g., Davidson, 1978; Straus, Gelles, & Steinmetz, 1980). The earliest recognition of the partner violence problem came decades, if not centuries, earlier (Davidson, 1978; Mowrer, 1938). As with many good ideas, however, once the prevention idea arrived it quickly took off. Now partner violence prevention programs occur in hundreds of communities and there are national organizations like the Family Violence Prevention Fund that are devoted to this task.

Yet, fundamental questions remain unanswered about partner violence prevention programs. There is already considerable similarity in both process and content among most partner violence prevention programs (e.g., Foshee, Bauman, Helms, Koch, & Linder, 1998; Jaffe et al., 1992; Weisz & Black, 2001). But does this similarity reflect a maturity of the field or pressure from communities to respond immediately to the partner violence problem and pressure from the scholarship system to publish quickly? Most existing evaluations are limited to studies examining the effectiveness of a single program. A few reviews exist of this research (e.g., Hamby, 1998), but these often focus on summarizing and evaluating existing studies. This paper will adopt a broader perspective. Instead of reviewing specific programs, the focus will be on issues relevant for a coherent program of partner violence prevention research. These include issues of the appropriate scope, format, audience, setting, and mechanics of partner violence prevention. In other words, questions of "who," "what," "when," "where," and "how" partner violence prevention should be conducted. Table 1 summarizes these questions, which are explored in more detail.

WHO SHOULD BE THE FOCUS
OF PARTNER VIOLENCE PREVENTION?

There is evidence that various partner violence prevention programs, most targeting school-aged youth, are at least somewhat effective in re-

TABLE 1. Summary of Questions for a Coherent Partner Violence Prevention Program

Who should be the focus of partner violence prevention?

(1). Are targeted or universal programs more effective?
(2). How do macrosocial programs, aimed at entire communities or societies, affect the outcomes of microsocial programs, which focus on individuals or couples?
(3). What programs are most cost-effective?
(4). Do some communities have characteristics that make targeted, universal, microsocial, or macrosocial programs more appropriate for them?

What should be the focus of partner violence prevention?

(1). Should programs be general and focus on more than one type of violence or even other social problems, or should they be specific to partner violence?
(2). Should programs focus on increasing protective factors or decreasing risk factors?

When in the lifespan should partner violence prevention be offered?

(1). Partner violence is clearly associated with youth, but what age is the best age to start prevention programs?
(2). Are there developmental milestones, such as engagement or marriage, where prevention should also be targeted?
(3). Would it be of any benefit to offer prevention programs later in life for any subset of the population?

Where are the best settings to offer partner violence prevention?

(1). What is the most appropriate setting for partner violence prevention programs?
(2). Are there advantages to schools, military bases, community centers, churches, health agencies, or other sites?
(3). How do issues of access, stigma, and impact vary across sites?

How should partner violence prevention programs be developed and evaluated?

(1). How should curricula take into considerations factors such as the importance of trauma history, cultural issues, and political issues such as regulations regarding sex education?
(2). How do measurement issues, such as accuracy of rates and exposure to related messages outside of the program under consideration, affect evaluations?
(3). How do program integrity, facilitator skill, and attendance affect evaluations of outcome?
(4). How do within-group differences, differences in pre-existing exposure to violence, and backlash affect evaluations of outcome?

ducing attitudes towards violence and violent behavior (e.g., Foshee et al., 1998; Jaffe et al., 1992; Markman, Renick, Floyd, Stanley, & Clements, 1993; Weisz & Black, 2001). To date, however, even the best evaluations of these programs have been limited to the comparison of a single, often new, program against no intervention or to even simpler single-group pretest-posttest designs (Hamby, 1998; O'Leary, Woodin, & Fritz, this volume). There is essentially no experimental data that directly address whether some types of prevention programs should be favored over others.

One of the big policy questions is whether programs should be targeted to specific risk groups among adults or be universal, that is, directed at everyone, especially perhaps at youthful populations such as students, active duty military, and newly married couples. (Targeted and universal prevention are also sometimes called "primary" and "secondary" prevention following Caplan, 1964.) It seems likely that both approaches will be needed for a social problem of the magnitude of partner violence, but it would be useful to have some guidance as to how to best combine efforts.

To fully understand how efforts can be combined, another dimension is needed as well (Godenzi & De Puy, 2001). Most evaluations have been done on programs that focus on individuals or couples, or operate at what can be called a "microsocial" level. These include programs that can be described as universal (all 6th graders, for example) or targeted (only children in some high risk category). Some programs, however, are intended to influence entire communities or societies and operate at "macrosocial" or "mesosocial" levels (Godenzi & De Puy, 2001). These usually fall in the universal category, but programs focusing on an entire high-risk community, such as an impoverished inner city area, could also be described as targeted. Microsocial programs, such as locally provided violence prevention curricula, are likely to take place in the context of macrosocial programs, such as public service campaigns and legal reform, that are also trying to reduce partner violence. Macro- social effects can come from not only orchestrated social efforts but also periodic media whirlwinds when celebrities are revealed to be in violent relationships with their partners (as either victim or perpetrator). Evaluations of mesosocial and macrosocial interventions are even rarer than evaluations of microsocial curricula, although they appear to at least increase helpseeking (cf. Hamby, 1998, for a review). These community-level events may have a profound impact on the results of programs that target individuals or groups.

We really do not have enough information to conclusively recommend whether universal or targeted approaches should receive more investment, but we can glean some hints from existing data and say with some certainty what sort of information would be needed to set evidence-based policy.

Relative Impact of Universal versus Targeted Programs

One of the most persuasive arguments for universal programs is the sheer number of individuals that are likely to be helped with universal approaches. Even modest effects, when they are applied to entire populations, can help very large numbers of people. On the other hand, targeted programs may more effectively prevent violence for the group that is in the most distress and perhaps has the greatest negative impact on the community. Surprisingly, formal comparisons of the two types of programs have not been conducted. Basic questions, such as whether the total amount of violence prevented differs for universal versus targeted programs, remain unanswered. Such studies are greatly needed.

Cost-Benefit Analyses

What is also missing from these considerations, from a policy perspective, is an estimate of costs. Two estimates are needed. One is an estimate of the relative costs of universal versus targeted programs. On a per-person basis, targeted programs will almost always be more expensive than universal programs. Targeted programs typically offer more labor-intensive services, such as individual or small group sessions and home visits. Targeted programs also often use providers with specialized training, who are costlier. Universal programs often make use of existing personnel, such as teachers, to implement programs and hence incur fewer direct labor charges. Nonetheless, if targeting can be done with a high degree of accuracy, targeted programs can still be more cost effective than universal programs. As with other program aspects, there have been no formal comparisons of the costs of universal versus targeted partner violence prevention programs. In fact, finding any information on the costs of administering prevention programs is difficult.

The other type of estimate that is needed to knowledgeably establish policy is an estimate of the costs of prevention versus the long-term costs of partner violence. Here more information is available, and existing data suggest that prevention is very inexpensive compared to the costs of intervening after the fact. There have been more formal analyses of the costs of violence than there have been of the savings associated with prevention. The figures are alarmingly high. For example, researchers in British Columbia, Canada, estimated that violence against women costs that province of 3.7 million people over $385 million dollars annually in law enforcement, lost work for victims, and interventions for victims, children, and offenders (Kerr & McLean, 1996). They were unable to quantify other significant monetary costs such as emergency medical care that would clearly add significantly to this figure. Lloyd (2002) offered an estimate of $273 million per year in direct costs of partner violence to the U.S. Department of Defense. These costs include diminished readiness, dismissal and training of replacement personnel, victim assistance, and intervention. Other effects, such as long-term intergenerational effects, are exceedingly difficult to quantify in terms of monetary costs but would surely bring these figures much higher.

Preventing partner violence also appears to be cost effective, although existing data are limited. Clark, Biddle, and Martin (2002) have recently calculated a cost-benefit analysis for the 1994 Violence Against Women Act (VAWA). VAWA spent $1.6 billion on various programs over five years, some of which were prevention programs (it was not possible to separate prevention from other programs). During this same period, they calculated that reductions in victimization, using National Criminal Victimization Survey data, saved $16.4 billion. Clark et al. do not consider factors besides increases in interventions and services. Some of this reduction in victimization, however, is probably due to an improving economy (Blumstein & Rosenfeld, 1999; Horton, 2002) and a reduction in the number of marriages (Dugan, Nagin, & Rosenfeld, 1999) during this same time period. Such factors can reduce stress and access (and hence violence) independently of VAWA programs. Nonetheless, even if VAWA accounted for only 10% of this reduction in victimization, Clark and her colleagues still found that the monetary benefits of the program outweighed the costs, and that less tangible benefits from reduction in distress, which are hard to quantify, provide additional support for prevention.

There do not seem to be studies of partner violence that directly compared the costs and potential savings of specific prevention programs, but a few well-done studies of this type have been done in other prevention fields. One such study examined the cost of preventing child maltreatment in Colorado (Gould & O'Brien, 1995). It was estimated that child maltreatment incurs direct annual costs of over $190 million dollars and further indirect costs of $212 million, for a total annual cost of over $403 million dollars related to child maltreatment in 1995. Gould and O'Brien suggest that an expanded targeted prevention program involving home visits for high-risk children could be implemented at a cost of about $32 million per year or about $2,000 per family. They indicate that the direct savings in foster care placements alone would be approximately $1.4 million dollars per year, even allowing for the fact that some (4%) of these children would probably end up in foster care anyway (Gould & O'Brien, 1995).

Community Culture

Another consideration when choosing universal versus targeted prevention programs, or between microsocial and macrosocial programs, is the culture of the community for which one proposes to intervene. One downside of targeted prevention programs is that they can be potentially stigmatizing if other members of a community become aware that an individual has been labeled high-risk. This is perhaps one reason why so many more universal programs exist in settings such as schools and military bases that are close knit and characterized by frequent group contact.

WHAT SHOULD BE THE FOCUS OF PARTNER VIOLENCE PREVENTION CURRICULA?

General versus Specific Programs

The other big policy question that follows from the developmental arc of aggression is whether prevention programs should be *general* and focus on more than one problem of youth or *specific* and focus on separate issues in separate programs.

Pros of General Programs. Many of the institutions that are likely to implement large-scale prevention programs, including schools, military bases, and community centers, have primary purposes other than the prevention of partner violence or other interpersonal or health problems. These institutions may not realistically have the time or resources to implement distinct curricula for every significant problem behavior. Professionals working with youth raised this issue during focus groups on partner violence prevention in Switzerland (De Puy & Hamby, 2003) and by advocates trying to gain access to school settings (Meyer & Stein, 2001). Further, many prevention programs include similar components such as communication skills and coping strategies and use similar instructional methods such as role-play and videos. This is true not only of partner violence prevention programs but also of prevention programs on numerous other topics such as school violence and substance abuse. Oftentimes, the most specific content is on risks and warning signs, and some research suggests such content is less effective than that which teaches skills (Hamby, 1998). So one question that should be addressed head on is whether it is worth it to develop programs for specific issues or whether the emphasis should be on general, topic-spanning interventions. Although such programs remain rare, there have been some preliminary efforts to address substance abuse and violent behavior in a single program for preschool children (Dubas, Lynch, Galano, Geller, & Hunt, 1998), and one project that suggested that a behavioral couples therapy program that targeted substance abusing partners also helped reduce domestic violence (O'Farrell, Van Hutton, & Murphy, 1999).

Unfortunately, it seems likely that the one of the main reasons that there are so many specific programs and so few general ones is because of the fragmentation among and within the various social and health sciences. Not only is there relatively little communication among psychologists, health providers, educators, and other human service professionals, but even within these fields there is isolation within subdisciplines and specialty areas (Hamby & Finkelhor, 2000). Disciplinary isolation and even "turf" issues minimize interest in analyses of whether these programs should be continued separately or not. More interdisciplinary, integrative work could answer key questions in this field.

Pros of Specific Programs. Nonetheless, there are important arguments to be made in favor of a specific approach to partner violence prevention. The basic question is whether there are issues unique to partner violence that cannot be addressed in more general anti-violence curricula. I believe the answer to that question is yes.

There are two different distinctions that can be made. First, there is the distinction between forms of intimate violence versus other interpersonal violence. Victims of all forms of intimate violence, including partner violence, sexual assault, child abuse, and elder abuse, share features that are not found among victims of assault by strangers. These include unique aspects of power, access, and betrayal (Hamby, 2004). Because of role relationships and the structure of families, victims of intimate assault may lack the power to respond in ways that are available to victims of stranger assault. Regarding partner violence specifically, men are, on average, over 30 pounds heavier, 5 inches taller (National Center for Health Statistics, 1994), and possess 50% more upper body and 30% more lower body strength than the average woman (Powers & Howley, 1997). This physical advantage is one reason why partner assaults of women are more likely to lead to injury than partner assaults of men (Stets & Straus, 1990; Tjaden & Thoennes, 2000). Further, despite strides towards more egalitarian relationships, male partners still typically earn more money and exercise more influence in most relationships (Fox & Murray, 2000; U.S. Census Bureau, 2001).

Known perpetrators often have frequent access to their victims. The repeated nature of partner violence, family violence, bullying, and gang violence is thought to be one of the most traumagenic features of these forms of violence (Banyard & Hamby, 1996). Access to victims exists on a continuum. Some perpetrators can have extensive access to victims. Regarding prevention, the most noteworthy situations are regular access through institutional contact such as schools and military bases. Intimate perpetrators, however, often have almost unlimited access to the victim. In particular, intimate partners are much more likely to have frequent private contact with their partners. Regarding betrayal, the intimate perpetrator violates not only norms for civil behavior but also personal bonds of trust (Hamby, 2004). It may be difficult for partners to reconcile the violence with what otherwise seems to be a loving and trusting relationship.

At a still greater level of specificity, there are unique dynamics associated with partner violence, even in comparison to other forms of intimate violence. Two of the most important are the particular vulnerabilities and trauma associated with sexual violence and the effect of gender roles on dating violence. Sexual assault has a number of unique harmful consequences, such as unwanted pregnancy, sexually transmitted diseases, and later sexual disorders. Contrary to some popular conceptions, most sexual assault is perpetrated by individuals known to the victim, including a significant percentage committed by spouses (Rennison, 2001b). Romantic relationships also have many unique characteristics that will not be addressed in curricula that focus on peer relationships. Teens will often accept things from boyfriends/girlfriends they would not from other peers. There is social pressure to be in a relationship and avoid terminating romantic relationships that does not exist for peer relationships (e.g., Hamby & Koss, 2003).

While I am drawing on existing information to postulate these differences, the question of whether general versus specific programs should be employed could be much more directly addressed through carefully designed research. For example, outcome evaluations of both types of programs could include questions on all of the major health behaviors that are targeted by prevention programs. It is not unreasonable to speculate that such surveys might discover, for instance, that improving communication skills in intimate relationships might affect condom use and hence help reduce sexually transmitted diseases, or that peer violence prevention programs would also reduce rates of partner violence. It is also possible that such spillover effects are minimal, or that they may apply to some behaviors but not others. For example, it might be possible to address various forms of acting out in a single program but not passive behaviors such as poor diet. This information would make it possible to craft evidence-based decisions regarding which problem behaviors can be addressed through omnibus efforts and which require special programming.

Increase Protective Factors or Decrease Risk Factors?

Another, related way of conceptualizing the content of prevention programs is to divide them between those that try to increase protective factors versus those that aim to reduce risk factors. A partner violence example of increasing a protective factor is teaching conflict resolution skills. An example of reducing a risk factor is teaching young people to avoid committed relationships with controlling and jealous individuals or to minimize such behavior themselves. This is related to the general versus specific dimension because many of the "general" elements turn out to be those that teach protective factors, such as teaching communication, conflict resolution, or social skills. A review of partner violence prevention research suggests that programs that focus on protective factors are more effective than programs that focus on risk factors alone (Hamby, 1998; O'Leary et al., this volume). Once again, though, this conclusion must be tempered by limitations in existing knowledge. For one, this distinction is not hard and fast, as many partner violence curricula, for example "Safe Dates" (Foshee et al., 1998), have elements that could be framed either way. For example, are segments on gender roles focusing on protective factors by encouraging healthy gender roles or are they focusing on risk factors by warning about negative gender stereotypes? Additionally, many of the better violence prevention programs include considerable material on both protective and risk factors and there have been no curriculum analyses so it is difficult to tell which elements are most responsible for observed changes. Outcome studies that manipulate the elements of curricula are needed to identify the best approach.

WHEN IN THE LIFESPAN SHOULD PARTNER VIOLENCE PREVENTION BE OFFERED?

Partner aggression has a well-established developmental arc–partner violence is much more common in late adolescence and young adulthood than it is at other developmental periods. Rates of partner violence are at least 2 to 3 times higher in this age group than among older adults (e.g., Office of Juvenile Justice & Delinquency Prevention, 2000;

O'Leary et al., this volume; Rennison, 2001a). Other behaviors that society tries to prevent are also more common among youth: substance abuse (Grant, 1996), risky sexual behavior (Abma, Chandra, Mosher, Peterson, & Piccinino, 1997), suicidality (Kessler, Borges, & Walter, 1999), and other interpersonal violence (Pastore & Maguire, 2003) are examples. All of these can be loosely grouped under the rubric of "acting out," which is considered one of the more primitive and less successful forms of coping (American Psychiatric Association [APA], 1994; Vaillant, 2000). Perhaps even other youth-associated problems such as eating disorders (APA, 1994) could be included in this classification. While of course all of these phenomena persist into middle age and beyond for a subset of the population, rates are significantly higher in the age range of roughly 15 to 29 year olds.

In contrast, there are a number of other problematic behaviors that are not associated with this developmental stage. Those that receive considerable attention and monetary investment from prevention experts include lack of exercise and other contributors to obesity (Centers for Disease Control and Prevention [CDC], 2003; Mokdad et al., 2003) and neglecting age-appropriate screening tests for cancer and other illnesses (CDC, 1989, 2003). These problems are often life-long and in many cases worsen with age. Unlike violence, these are often problems of withdrawal and passivity rather than acting out. Finally, the last major arena that receives the attention of prevention experts is developmental events such as terrorist attacks and natural disasters. The goal of prevention efforts in these cases is usually to prevent or diminish the severity of posttraumatic stress symptoms. Because the targets of terrorist attacks are often the general population and natural disasters have random targets, exposure to such events is less tied to developmental stages. Nonetheless, exposure to some of these events, or especially to the aftermath of these events, may have some developmental relationship as disaster workers and military personnel are younger than the general population of adults.

Most existing prevention programs are aimed at young people and so the field is currently using one of the best documented risk factors to target programs. This is probably one of the smartest steps prevention specialists have taken to date. There are still unanswered questions though. What age is the best age to start? Are there developmental milestones, such as engagement or marriage, where prevention should also be targeted? Would it be of any benefit to offer prevention programs later in life for any subset of the population? These questions are tied to the question of what setting is most appropriate for partner violence prevention programs.

WHERE ARE THE BEST SETTINGS TO OFFER PARTNER VIOLENCE PREVENTION?

What is the most appropriate institutional setting for partner violence prevention programs? Are there advantages to schools, military bases, community centers, churches, health agencies, or other sites? O'Leary et al. (this volume) have noted that motivation is a key factor in seeking prevention, and one key variable that these sites vary on is the voluntariness of participation. Different forms of motivation may have different results. For example, I once helped facilitate a prevention program for engaged couples that took place in a local church. The minister referred all couples who wanted to marry in that church. Although the program was voluntary, his endorsement led to a very high participation rate. Again, as with these other issues, this is a variable that could be formally manipulated in well-designed research.

The most appropriate site can vary across communities, as well. In many communities, schools are becoming increasingly regimented by the demands of achievement testing and also by the politics of dealing with nontraditional subjects in school settings. Time is a major issue in convincing schools to adopt a curriculum in addition to these demands (Meyer & Stein, 2001). Nonetheless, public schools are still favored in the U.S. because they provide the easiest access to the broadest segment of the youth population (although children in private, parochial, and home school settings are missed with this approach). There is also considerable variability across countries as well. School structures can vary substantially, and in some countries more of the population has access to community centers or local health agencies than is typically true in the U.S., providing possible alternatives to school settings that would still reach a substantial portion of youth (De Puy & Hamby, 2003).

HOW SHOULD PARTNER VIOLENCE PREVENTION PROGRAMS BE DEVELOPED AND EVALUATED?

Beyond establishing broad policy guidelines for the "who," "what," "when," and "where" of partner violence prevention are a plethora of nitty-gritty issues of methodology and analysis. These need to be addressed to put prevention outcome research on a par with the best treatment outcome research. Elsewhere in this volume, O'Leary et al. have identified several important criteria that future projects should be evaluated on. I will reiterate them here but not comment on them further.

They have cited: ceiling effects, effects of facilitator enthusiasm (or lack thereof), haphazard curriculum assembly, need for curriculum analysis, program brevity, no analyses of needed program length, need for more behavioral measures, longer follow-ups, and need to consider the appropriate unit of analysis in choice of statistics. There are a few additional criteria that also need consideration.

Curriculum Issues

Content Should Reflect Knowledge of Risk Factors. Curricula should be much more closely based on the existing knowledge about risk factors for violence. There are a number of risk factors that might be more thoroughly addressed by most curricula, but I will mention one of the strongest and best-documented risk factor that receives essentially no attention in any prevention curricula I have seen: trauma history.

Learning to cope successfully with trauma histories is surely one of the single largest factors in reducing partner violence, both in terms of perpetration and (re-)victimization. Probably 1/4 to 1/3 of any adult group has some sort of trauma history, and these are conservative estimates because comprehensive assessments of all major forms of trauma are rarely done (Hamby & Finkelhor, 2000). Recent longitudinal data suggest that a childhood history of abuse and exposure to domestic violence are two of the largest risks for later partner violence (Ehrensaft, Cohen, Brown, Smailes, Chen, & Johnson, 2003). It is also noteworthy that trauma histories are closely associated with other acting out problems too, such as substance abuse, suicidality, and eating disorders (e.g., Kilpatrick, Ruggiero, Acierno, Saunders, Resnick, & Best, 2003; Mussell, Binford, & Fulkerson, 2000). At most, current programs recommend counseling and provide numbers of local providers. This issue could be addressed in a prevention program using a cognitive-behavioral/psychoeducational framework that is consistent with other modules. Many counselors recommend the cognitive-behavioral approach to trauma symptoms. Programs could include coping techniques to deal with stress and trauma, such as grounding, self-talk, and expressive writing, in addition to problem solving and communication skills. They could address issues of self-blame, victim-blame, and the intergenerational cycle of violence.

Community and Cultural Issues. There are any number of issues that might need to be addressed in specific communities. This includes not only content but also instructional techniques. For example, in our Swiss project, we had a high percentage of immigrant youth. While they were fluent in spoken French, many of them were uncomfortable with the writing exercises and we revised or omitted many of these from the original curriculum (DePuy & Hamby, 2003). As another example, in a prevention program with Apache high school students, we had to adapt most of the class-wide public-speaking exercises into small group or individual exercises. While some Apache youth were comfortable with public speaking, it was perceived by some as behavior more appropriate for elders or others with authority.

Inclusion of Family Members. Some programs are beginning to incorporate parents and children, but this is still rarely emphasized and could be an important key to maintaining the gains shown immediately upon program completion.

Realities of Regulations. Over the years, a number of state and Federal regulations have defined or restricted what many professionals may share with youth. This includes information about abortion and sex education. For example, in North Carolina, sex education must be restricted to abstinence only programs. In some counties, this has been interpreted to mean that sexual assault prevention is not consistent with this regulation. In at least one county, however, anti-violence advocates have persuaded school personnel that "don't have forced sex" is consistent with the abstinence message of "don't have sex" (B. Massey, MSW, personal communication, April, 2002). While the logic of this argument may be awkward, it also reflects the political realities that many agencies face.

Measurement Issues

Precise Incidence and Prevalence Rates for Violence. While it is generally acknowledged that existing self-report methods identify more cases of partner violence than official reports, more needs to be done to improve assessment. Techniques such as audio-enhanced computer-assisted self interview (audio-CASI) have been shown to increase the disclosure of violence and other sensitive behaviors in a number of studies (e.g., Percy & Mayhew, 1997; Turner et al., 1998). Like many batterers evaluation studies, prevention outcome research needs to use existing official data as a supplement to self-report. This is sometimes done in studies of school violence, where data on suspensions and other school incidents are often available. Partner violence programs that take place in institutional settings such as military bases and schools may have better knowledge of instances than is true of the general population. Accurate cost-benefit analyses cannot be conducted without accurate data on rates, and the more error in measures of violence, the more difficult it will be to observe program effects.

Exposure to the Program's Message Outside of the Program. Anti-violence messages come from many sources, including the media, health and human service providers, and community organizations, and it is generally not possible to totally control exposure to these messages. Thus, it would make sense to measure them. Participants in both the experimental and control groups could be asked, at least at post-test, whether they have heard relevant news stories, seen public service announcements, or become aware of community services during the course of the evaluation. This would be particularly important if a well-publicized incident occurred during an evaluation, such as a domestic violence murder or trial or news of the alleged involvement of a celebrity in a domestic violence incident (as either victim or perpetrator). Measure of exposure and consideration of history would give a much truer idea of the difference between the experimental and "control" group.

Methodological Issues

Manipulation Checks. Some years ago, therapy outcome researchers discovered that therapists did not always stick to the orientation or intervention to which they had been assigned in treatment outcome studies. The majority of prevention researchers have yet to realize that their facilitators may need monitoring as well, so that more accurate measures of dose and intervention take place. Of course, facilitators should not be required to read the manual aloud word-for-word and ruin with a stilted delivery what might have worked with a natural speaking presentation. Nonetheless, researchers should assess what is said, what exercises are done, and what stimulus materials are used. In my experience with prevention specialists, many respond to what they perceive as participants' boredom, lack of comprehension, and time pressures in their schedule by altering or shortening stimulus materials and videos. This is especially true outside of controlled outcome studies, where another popular option is to simply pick and choose 2 or 3 elements from a program that fit a teacher's interest and time. Video or audio-taping, facilitator self-report, or periodic observations could all be used to monitor program delivery.

Practice. Another lesson that can be taken from therapy outcome studies is that novice therapists are almost always worse than experienced therapists (e.g., Huppert, Bufka, Barlow, Gorman, Shear, & Woods, 2001). In fact, this is one of the most reliable therapist characteristics that affect outcome. Many published prevention evaluations, even for successful, well-validated studies like SAFE DATES, appear to be the first or one of the first implementations of these programs (SAFE DATES ©1994, the same year that the implementation that is the basis of the evaluation took place; Foshee et al., 1998). Further, very little is usually said about the training in the specific curriculum or the general teaching and/or counseling experience of the individuals who deliver the program. The Swiss professionals in our focus groups were surprised that we were considering evaluating the first implementation of a partner violence prevention program and quickly informed us of their preference to have at least one complete trial run prior to any formal evaluation (DePuy & Hamby, 2003).

Choice of Facilitator. Often, financial considerations lead people to use existing staff, such as teachers, to deliver prevention programs. Teachers are likely to be more familiar with their audience but perhaps less experienced in the topic area or with the challenges of publicly presenting what can be sensitive material. In one study of a sexual abuse prevention program, no differences in efficacy were found between teachers and expert facilitators (Hazzard, Kleemeier, & Webb, 1990). It should be noted, however, that in this study, all facilitators received extensive training before implementing the program, and the teachers had the advantage of delivering the program to smaller groups than the experts. More work in this area needs to be done.

Attendance and Dose. One basic dose issue is determining the program length needed to observe an effect (Meyer & Stein, 2001; O'Leary et al., this volume). Attendance is another important factor in assessing dose and response. Studies of batterers intervention suggest that the same group who are most likely to benefit from treatment–employed, married men with higher levels of education–are also the group most likely to complete treatment once they start it (Hamby, 1998). Poor school attendance is correlated with a host of family and adjustment problems. Consequently, prevention programs that are offered in the schools may less often reach those who need it most.

Analytical Issues

Within-Group Differences. Another extremely important question is: "Who gets better in prevention programs?" One problem in documenting improvement is the ceiling effects typically observed in attitude reporting. The majority of young people, typically over 70% or 80%, report virtually "ideal" attitudes in support of nonviolence. A clear majority also reports no violent behavior (although some of these are probably failing to disclose their true attitudes and behavior). Although nonviolence describes the majority of youths' attitudes and behaviors, there is still a large group that has room for improvement. But who among the violent respond to prevention programs? Is it the 30% or more who have used (or experienced) mild physical aggression, or the much smaller portion (under 10%) who have used or experienced severe physical aggression or sexual aggression (cf. Foshee et al., 1996; Straus, Hamby, Boney-McCoy, & Sugarman, 1996 for rates)?

Once again, the existing partner violence prevention literature cannot answer this question. But the history of research on other interventions suggests that it is more likely that we are reaching the mild aggressors and not the severe ones (e.g., Mohr, 1995; Siqueland et al., 2002). Although there is little research on the "natural history" of partner violence (to borrow a term from medicine), what does exist suggests that perpetrators of severe and frequent violence are more likely to persist than perpetrators of minor and infrequent violence (e.g., Woffordt, Mihalic, & Menard, 1994). Treatment outcome literature has generally shown that people with multiple problems or disorders are harder to treat than those with one diagnosis. What we know about severe batterers suggests that the majority have other significant problems, including substance abuse, problems with violence in other relationships, personality disorders such as antisocial and borderline personalities, and other mental health issues (e.g., Holtzworth-Munroe & Stuart, 1994). It seems likely that this group is less likely to respond to a prevention program, whether universal or targeted.

Measure Prevention or Intervention? True prevention usually refers to eliminating a problem before it occurs. For example, universal vaccination prevents childhood diseases before they occur. Targeted or secondary prevention programs usually identify a high-risk group based on one problem and then try to keep them from developing other, related problems. An example of this type of program is Head Start, which uses low socioeconomic status and other factors to identify children who may develop problems in school and tries to increase school readiness before they enter kindergarten.

These make nice, clean examples because they take advantage of fairly well-defined developmental milestones that define onset (i.e., children are vaccinated before there is much chance they will acquire a disease and given extra instruction before they begin regular school). The developmental issues regarding partner violence prevention are more complex. Partner violence rates dramatically increase in high school and remain high throughout young adulthood, then tapering off. It is thought to be relatively uncommon for someone to suddenly begin using violence in their 30s or beyond. So in that sense it is associated with a fairly distinct developmental stage, and that is one reason why it is of such interest to institutions dealing with adolescents and young adults such as schools, universities, and the military.

On the other hand, one of the main reasons for this developmental timing is the onset of puberty and the beginning of dating relationships. As is well known by anyone with much exposure to pre-pubertal youth, those approaching puberty usually perceive dating relationships very differently compared to those experiencing it. This period of life also corresponds to major cognitive changes for many youth, as many achieve the ability to use hypothetical and abstract thinking about the time they reach puberty. Cognitive abilities influence the way that children interpret violence events (Buckley, 2000). These cognitive skills are also crucial for predicting possible alternative scenarios that result from various conflict resolution strategies and other elements that are key to avoiding violence. As far as I am aware, no one has attempted to implement a partner violence program with elementary school youth. There are violence prevention programs for this age group, but they teach skills that are considerably more general and basic and may well not be seen to apply to romantic relationships.

As a result, partner violence prevention programs must deal with the fact that many individuals in their programs are already violent. Strictly speaking, we are examining intervention effects with these individuals, not prevention. True prevention effects would involve monitoring the majority who are nonviolent at the time of the program and seeing if they maintain this nonviolence at greater rates than a control group who does not receive the program. Of course, both prevention and intervention effects are desirable, but they should be monitored separately in outcome studies.

Backlash. Even the above framework, which calls for separate monitoring of intervention and prevention effects, is overly simple. Another area that needs more attention is a close examination of whether prevention programs are ever iatrogenic, and if so, for whom. Of course, it is unavoidable that the occasional participant will experience more victimization or perpetrate more violence after a prevention program than prior to it, just due to random life events or perhaps more disclosure at follow-up than during the pretest.

While few evaluators have considered the possibility of backlash, Jaffe et al. (1992) found that a small subgroup of students, mostly males, reported more negative attitudes towards partner violence after a prevention program than before it. What needs to be determined is whether there are more individuals with worsening attitudes in program groups compared to control groups. This calls for analytic strategies that look at individual change patterns and not just mean group differences.

CONCLUSIONS

The "why" of partner violence prevention is readily apparent, with lifetime rates of partner violence victimization in the 25% to 35% range or perhaps even higher (Straus & Gelles, 1990; Tjaden & Thoennes, 2000). There is a strong need for partner violence prevention, especially in the late adolescent and young adult population, where rates of partner violence are very high. The answers to most other questions about the science of partner violence prevention research are virtually unknown. There are a number of broad policy issues that would benefit from studies comparing different approaches to prevention. These include the question of whether partner violence prevention should be universal, targeted, or both, whether partner violence prevention should be included in general curricula or be taught in specialized programs, and whether partner violence prevention instruction should focus more on protective or risk factors. Research also needs to explore not only which types of programs are more effective but also identify the reasons why some content is more helpful than others. These are questions with empirical answers that could be answered with a sound partner violence prevention research program. To date, Federal and other funding agencies have made little effort to answer these questions. The answers have the potential to improve the lives of thousands of people.

REFERENCES

Abma, J., Chandra, A., Mosher, W., Peterson, L., & Piccinino, L. (1997). *Fertility, family planning, and women's health: New data from the 1995 National Survey of Family Growth* (Vital Health Statistics Series 23 No 19). Washington, DC: National Center for Health Statistics.

American Psychiatric Association. (1994). *Diagnostic and statistical manual of mental disorders* (4th ed.). Washington, DC: Author.

Banyard, V. L., & Hamby, S. L. (1996, August). The experience of powerlessness and consequences of child sexual abuse. In S. L. Hamby (Chair), *Theorizing about gender socialization and power in family violence*. Symposium conducted at the American Psychological Association Annual Meeting, Toronto, Ontario.

Blumstein, A., & Rosenfeld, R. (1999). Trends in rates of violence in the U.S.A. *Studies on Crime and Crime Prevention, 8*(2), 139-167.

Buckley, M. A. (2000). Cognitive-developmental considerations in violence prevention and intervention. *Professional School Counseling, 4*, 60-71.

Caplan, G. (1964). *Principles of preventive psychiatry*. New York: Basic Books.

Centers for Disease Control and Prevention. (1989). Current trends in pap smear screening–Behavioral Risk Factor Surveillance System, 1988. *Morbidity and Mortality Weekly Report, 38*(45), 777-779.

Centers for Disease Control and Prevention. (2003). *Behavioral Risk Factor Surveillance System survey data*. Atlanta, GA: Author. Retrieved January 1, 2004 from, http://apps.nccd.cdc.gov/brfss/page.asp?yr=2002&state=US&cat=WH#WH

Clark, K. A., Biddle, A. K., & Martin, S. L. (2002). A cost-benefit analysis of the Violence Against Women Act of 1994. *Violence Against Women, 8*(4), 417-428.

Davidson, T. (1978). *Conjugal crime: Understanding and changing the wifebeating pattern*. New York: Hawthorn Books, Inc.

De Puy, J., & Hamby, S. L. (2003, June). *A culture of peace and equality in intimate relationships: Bringing teen dating violence prevention/promotion of healthy relationships to Switzerland*. Presented at the UNESCO Conference on Intercultural Education, Jyvaskyla, Finland.

Dubas, J. S., Lynch, K. B., Galano, J., Geller, S., & Hunt, D. (1998). Preliminary evaluation of a resiliency-based preschool substance abuse and violence prevention project. *Journal of Drug Education, 28*(3), 235-255.

Dugan, L., Nagin, D., & Rosenfeld, R. (1999). Explaining the decline in intimate partner homicide: The effects of changing domesticity, women's status, and domestic violence resources. *Homicide Studies, 3*, 187-214.

Ehrensaft, M. K., Cohen, P., Brown, J., Smailes, E., Chen, H., & Johnson, J. G. (2003). Intergenerational transmission of partner violence: A 20-year prospective study. *Journal of Consulting and Clinical Psychology, 71*, 741-753.

Foshee, V. A., Bauman, K. E., Helms, R. W., Koch, G. G., & Linder, G. F. (1998). An evaluation of Safe Dates, an adolescent dating violence prevention program. *American Journal of Public Health, 88*, 45-50.

Foshee, V. A., Linder, G., Bauman, K., Langwick, S., Arriaga, X., Heath, J. et al. (1996). The Safe Dates Project: Theoretical basis, evaluation design, and selected baseline findings. *American Journal of Preventive Medicine, 12*, 39-47.

Fox, G. L., & Murry, V. M. (2000). Gender and families: Feminist perspectives and family research. *Journal of Marriage and the Family, 62*(4), 1160-1172.

Godenzi, A., & De Puy, J. (2001). Overcoming boundaries: A cross-cultural inventory of primary prevention programs against wife abuse and child abuse. *The Journal of Primary Prevention, 21*, 455-475.

Gould, M. S., & O'Brien, T. (1995). *Child maltreatment in Colorado: The value of prevention and the cost of failure to prevent*. Denver, CO: Colorado Children's Trust Fund.

Grant, B. F. (1996). Prevalence and correlates of drug use and DSM-IV drug dependence in the United States: Results of the National Longitudinal Alcohol Epidemiologic Survey. *Journal of Substance Abuse, 8*(2), 195-210.

Hamby, S. L. (1998). Prevention and intervention of partner violence. In L. Williams & J. Jasinski (Eds.), *Partner violence: A comprehensive review of 20 years of research* (pp. 210-258). Newbury Park, CA: Sage Publications.

Hamby, S. L. (2004). The spectrum of victimization and the implications for health. In Kendall-Tackett, K. (Ed), *Health consequences of abuse in the family: A clinical guide for practice.* Washington, DC: American Psychological Association (pp. 7-27).

Hamby, S. L., & Finkelhor, D. (2000). The victimization of children: Recommendations for assessment and instrument development. *Journal of the American Academy of Child and Adolescent Psychiatry, 39*(7), 829-840.

Hamby, S. L., & Koss, M. P. (2003). Shades of gray: A qualitative study of terms used in the measurement of sexual victimization. *Psychology of Women Quarterly, 27,* 243-255.

Hazzard, A. P., Kleemeier, C. P., & Webb, C. (1990). Teacher versus expert presentations of sexual abuse prevention programs. *Journal of Interpersonal Violence, 5*(1), 23-36.

Holtzworth-Munroe, A. & Stuart, G. L. (1994). Typologies of male batterers: Three subtypes and the differences among them. *Psychological Bulletin, 116,* 476-497.

Horton, A. (2002). Violent crime: New evidence to consider. *Journal of Human Behavior for the Social Environment, 5*(2), 77-88.

Huppert, J. D., Bufka, L. F., Barlow, D. H., Gorman, J. M., Shear, M. K., & Woods, S. W. (2001). Therapists, therapist variables, and cognitive-behavioral therapy outcome in a multicenter trial for panic disorder. *Journal of Consulting and Clinical Psychology, 69*(5), 747-755.

Jaffe, P. G., Sudermann, M., Reitzel, D., & Killip, S. M. (1992). An evaluation of a secondary school primary prevention program on violence in intimate relationships. *Violence and Victims, 7*(2), 129-146.

Jones, L. E. (1991). The Minnesota School Curriculum Project: A statewide domestic violence prevention project in secondary schools. In B. Levy (Ed.), *Dating violence: Young women in danger* (pp. 258-266). Seattle, WA: Seal Press.

Kerr, R., & McLean, J. (1996). *Paying for violence: Some of the costs of violence against women in B.C.* Victoria, BC: British Columbia Ministry of Women's Equality.

Kessler, R. C., Borges, G., & Walters, E. E. (1999). Prevalence of and risk factors for lifetime suicide attempts in the National Comorbidity Survey. *Archives of General Psychiatry, 56*(7), 617-626.

Kilpatrick, D. G., Ruggiero, K. J., Acierno, R., Saunders, B. E., Resnick, H. S., & Best, C. L. (2003). Violence and risk of PTSD, major depression, substance abuse/dependence, and comorbidity: Results from the National Survey of Adolescents. *Journal of Consulting and Clinical Psychology, 71,* 692-700.

Lloyd, D. (2002, May). *Welcome and purpose of meeting.* Presented at the Department of Defense Maltreatment Prevention Symposium, Arlington, VA.

Markman, H. J., Renick, M. J., Floyd, F. J., Stanley, S. M., & Clements, M. (1993). Preventing marital distress through communication and conflict management training:

A 4- and 5-year follow-up. *Journal of Consulting and Clinical Psychology, 61,* 70-76.

Meyer, H., & Stein, N. (2001, July). *Relationship violence prevention education in schools: What's working, what's getting in the way, what might be some future directions.* Presented at the 7th International Family Violence Research Conference, Portsmouth, NH.

Mohr, D. C. (1995). Negative outcome in psychotherapy: A critical review. *Clinical Psychology: Science and Practice, 2,* 1-27.

Mokdad, A. H., Ford, E.S., Bowman, B. A., Dietz, W. H., Vinicor, F., Bales, V. S. et al. (2003). Prevalence of obesity, diabetes, and obesity-related health risk factors, 2001. *Journal of the American Medical Association, 289,* 76-79.

Mowrer, E. R. (1938). The trend and ecology of family disintegration in Chicago. *American Sociological Review, 3,* 344-353.

Mussell, M. P., Binford, R. B., & Fulkerson, J. A. (2000). Eating disorders: Summary of risk factors, prevention programming, and prevention research. *The Counseling Psychologist, 28*(6), 764-796.

National Center for Health Statistics. (1994). *National Health and Nutrition Survey data tables.* Hyattsville, MD: National Center for Health Statistics.

O'Farrell, T. J., Van Hutton, V., & Murphy, C. M. (1999). Domestic violence after alcoholism treatment: A two-year longitudinal study. *Journal of Studies on Alcohol, 60,* 317-321.

Office of Juvenile Justice & Delinquency Prevention (2000). *Children as victims: 1999 national report series (NCJ 180753).* Washington, DC: Author.

O'Leary, K. D., Woodin, E. M., & Fritz, P. T. (2006). Prevention of aggression in intimate partner relationships. *Journal of Aggression, Maltreatment and Trauma, 13*(3/4), 121-178.

Pastore, A. L., & Maguire, K. (Eds.) (2003, August). Percent distribution of total U.S. population and persons arrested for all offenses. *Sourcebook of Criminal Justice Statistics* [Online]. Retrieved December 30, 2003 from, http://www.albany.edu/sourcebook/1995/pdf/t44.pdf

Percy, A., & Mayhew, P. (1997). Estimating sexual victimization in a national survey: A new approach. *Studies on Crime and Prevention, 6*(2), 125-150.

Powers, S. K., & Howley, E. T. (1997). *Exercise physiology: Theory and application to fitness and performance* (3rd ed.). Dubuque, IA: Brown & Benchmark.

Rennison, C. M. (2001a). *Intimate partner violence and age of victim, 1993-1999 (NCJ 187635).* Washington, DC: Bureau of Justice Statistics.

Rennison, C. M. (2001b). *Criminal victimization 2000: Changes 1999-2000 with trends 1993-2000* (NCJ 187007). Washington, DC: Bureau of Justice Statistics, U.S. Department of Justice.

Siqueland, L., Crits, C. P., Gallop, R., Barber, J. P., Griffin, M. L., Thase, M. E. et al. (2002). Retention in psychosocial treatment of cocaine dependence: Predictors and impact on outcome. *American Journal on Addictions, 11*(1), 24-40.

Stets, J. E., & Straus, M. A. (1990). Gender differences in reporting marital violence and its medical and psychological consequences. In M. A. Straus & R. J. Gelles (Eds.), *Physical violence in American families: Risk factors and adaptations to violence in 8,145 families* (pp. 151-165). New Brunswick, NJ: Transaction.

Straus, M. A., & Gelles, R. J. (1990). *Physical violence in American families: Risk factors and adaptations to violence in 8,145 families.* New Brunswick, NJ: Transaction Publishers.

Straus, M. A., Gelles, R. J., & Steinmetz, S. K. (1980). *Behind closed doors: Violence in the American family.* New York: Doubleday.

Straus, M. A., Hamby, S. L., Boney-McCoy, S., & Sugarman, D. B. (1996). The Revised Conflict Tactics Scales (CTS2): Development and preliminary psychometric data. *Journal of Family Issues, 17,* 283-316.

Tjaden, P., & Thoennes, N. (2000). *Extent, nature, and consequences of intimate partner violence: Findings from the National Violence Against Women Survey.* Washington, DC: National Institutes of Justice.

Turner, C. F., Ku, L., Rogers, S. M., Lindberg, L. D., Pleck, J. H., & Sonenstein, F. L. (1998). Adolescent sexual behavior, drug use, and violence: Increased reporting with computer survey technology. *Science, 280,* 867-873.

U.S. Census Bureau. (2001, October 5). *Historical income tables–People.* U.S. Census Bureau. Retrieved February 13, 2002 from, http://www.census.gov/hhes/histinc/p38a.html

Vaillant, G. E. (2000). Adaptive mental mechanisms: Their role in a positive psychology. *American Psychologist, 55*(1), 89-98.

Violence Against Women Act of 1994, Title IV of the Violent Crime Control and Law Enforcement Act, Pub. L. No. 103-322.

Walther, D. J. (1986). Wife abuse prevention: Effects of information on attitudes of high school boys. *Journal of Primary Prevention, 7*(2), 84-90.

Weisz, A. N., & Black, B. M. (2001). Evaluating a sexual assault and dating violence prevention program for urban youths. *Social Work Research, 25,* 89-91.

Woffordt, S., Mihalic, D. E., & Menard, S. (1994). Continuities in marital violence. *Journal of Family Violence, 9,* 195-225.

doi:10.1300/J146v13n03_07

CHANGING THE WAYS COMMUNITIES SUPPORT FAMILIES TO PREVENT INTIMATE PARTNER VIOLENCE

Preventing Intimate Partner Violence: A Community Capacity Approach

Jay A. Mancini
John P. Nelson
Gary L. Bowen
James A. Martin

SUMMARY. Bringing together the energy, resources, creativity, and good will of citizens enhances community resilience. The shared responsibility and collective competence that emerge from community members banding together can be a powerful and ongoing positive influence on the quality of community life, including the relationships between intimate partners. We explore the importance that the community has for preventing intimate partner violence (IPV). We argue for active,

Address correspondence to: Jay A. Mancini, PhD, Department of Human Development, 303 Wallace Hall, Virginia Polytechnic Institute and State University, Blacksburg, VA 24061.

[Haworth co-indexing entry note]: "Preventing Intimate Partner Violence: A Community Capacity Approach." Mancini, Jay A. et al. Co-published simultaneously in *Journal of Aggression, Maltreatment & Trauma* (The Haworth Maltreatment & Trauma Press, an imprint of The Haworth Press, Inc.) Vol. 13, No. 3/4, 2006, pp. 203-227; and: *Prevention of Intimate Partner Violence* (ed: Sandra M. Stith) The Haworth Maltreatment & Trauma Press, an imprint of The Haworth Press, Inc., 2006, pp. 203-227. Single or multiple copies of this article are available for a fee from The Haworth Document Delivery Service [1-800-HAWORTH, 9:00 a.m. - 5:00 p.m. (EST). E-mail address: docdelivery@haworthpress.com].

network-oriented prevention efforts. We discuss key community principles and concepts (including a definition of the nature of community), explore a social organization perspective on communities, and present a theoretical approach to building community capacity. We posit implications for program development that include community as a place for prevention, a target for prevention, and as a force for prevention. Our implications for research include examining multiple community layers, the nexus of informal and formal social care systems, and contrasting extreme groups on pivotal social organization processes. doi:10.1300/J146v13n03_08 *[Article copies available for a fee from The Haworth Document Delivery Service: 1-800-HAWORTH. E-mail address: <docdelivery@haworthpress.com> Website: <http://www.HaworthPress.com>*

KEYWORDS. Intimate partner violence, community capacity theory, social networks, community development, prevention

Community resilience and the benefits a community provides to its residents can be enhanced by collective action, that is, by bringing together the energy, resources, creativity, and good will of citizens. The shared responsibility and collective competence that emerge from community members banding together can become a powerful and ongoing positive influence on the quality of community life, including the relationships between intimate partners. This community capacity for building an environment that supports children, youth, families, and adults can lead to the attainment of important community results, including safer neighborhoods, healthier children, and intimate partners who resolve issues without using violence.

We explore the importance that the community may have for preventing intimate partner violence (IPV). We reject reliance on passive, public-service-announcement approaches, and argue instead for active, network-oriented prevention efforts. We predicate our approach on the reality that humans are social beings and are influenced by social phenomena that include culture, norms, and community social organization. We discuss key community principles and concepts (including a definition of the nature of community), explore a social organization approach to communities, and present an approach to building community capacity. We posit implications for research and for program development.

Chaskin, Brown, Venkatesh, and Vidal (2001) raise the question, what is a community that "works"? Sampson (2001) asks, what are the collective processes that make for a healthy neighborhood environment? We ask, more specifically, what are the community elements that promote healthy relationships and minimize IPV, and what ongoing prevention systems can be put in place to provide community elements that make positive differences?

INTIMATE PARTNER VIOLENCE TRENDS

In 2001, approximately 588,490 U.S. women reported physical or sexual assault by intimates, and men were victims of about 103,220 violent crimes committed by an intimate partner (Rennison, 2003). Rates of IPV range from 1.8% to 14% in population-based studies, and up to 44% in health care settings (Jones et al., 1999; Tjaden & Thoennes, 2000). Lifetime estimates range up to 51%, with a typical range between 25% and 35% (Tjaden & Thoennes, 2000). Women experience significantly more violence from intimate partners than men do (Bachman, 1994; Tjaden & Thoennes). More than 25% of American married couples experience one or more incidents of IPV (Feld & Straus, 1989).

PROGRAM RESPONSES TO INTIMATE PARTNER VIOLENCE

Today's response to IPV is shaped by legal reforms over the past two decades and is characterized by comprehensive and aggressive law enforcement actions focused on offender accountability and on deterring offenders' behaviors. Nevertheless, incidence and prevalence data demonstrate that legal reform alone is not sufficient, and suggest that culture and community reform are necessary (Daro, Edleson, & Pinderhughes, 2004). The prevalence of attitudes and community norms that support violence against women, excusing violence as private or as deserved by the victim, remains one of the most distressing issues in efforts to stop IPV. Community education and media campaigns directed at changing attitudes and public opinion are the dominant community-based prevention strategies, and are largely ineffective in changing behavior because they tend to be passive, stand-alone interventions rather than part of a more comprehensive strategy (Snyder, 2001). An approach with greater potential to effect change involves the activities of formal and informal community networks.

Two decades ago, the Attorney General's Task Force on Family Violence recommended coordinated community responses to IPV and specified reforms in the law and the operations of the criminal justice system (Department of Justice, 1984). Unfortunately, although community-wide responses to IPV are strongly encouraged, they are rarely obtained. Often, communities merely respond to violence, rather than proactively structuring prevention initiatives, and coordination occurs across a limited set of formal community organizations, principally those representing the criminal justice system (Pence, 1983; Shepard, 1999). Generally excluded from coordinated community response models are formal community agencies such as healthcare, faith-based, or community organizations, and informal networks such as family, friends, neighbors, or work associates.

Wolfe and Jaffe (2003) and O'Leary, Woodin, and Fritz (this volume) review IPV and sexual assault prevention programs across the age continuum, from elementary-aged children to college students and young adults. While some prevention programs target high-risk groups, most prevention efforts are psychoeducational and target a broad population. Such programs focus on clarifying attitudes and behaviors and on offering positive norms and alternatives. Wolfe and Jaffe note that schools are the ideal venues for most of these primary prevention programs. In contrast, prevention strategies targeting adults are generally limited to media or public awareness campaigns–advertisements or public service announcements providing information on community resources.

These approaches are passive, less intensive, and lack focus. For instance, the National Violence Against Women Prevention Research Center (2002) found that current prevention programs are limited in scope; that programs target mostly females, without acknowledging the role males play in preventing violence against women; and that few programs focus on perpetrators. Most programs are nonstandardized, in-house initiatives that lack common components and substantive evaluation efforts. These findings illustrate the need for more systematic program evaluation as well as more development and dissemination of structured prevention programs.

There are few controlled-outcome studies of interpersonal violence prevention programs (O'Leary, Woodin, & Friz, this volume), and these studies focus on adolescent dating violence rather than on young adults or on married couples. Wolfe and Jaffe (2003) also note the meager amount of existing research and its narrow focus. O'Leary et al. review substance abuse prevention research, which is substantial, to identify potential links and lessons for intimate partner violence prevention programs. Their review shows that successful programs (a) target behavior rather than attitudes; (b) involve interactive components rather than didactic instruction; (c) include a cognitive or cognitive-behavioral orientation, especially social skills training and norms education; (d) consist of longer treatment and follow-up sessions instead of one-time programs; and (e) emphasize culturally appropriate programs.

Reviews of mass media education and awareness prevention campaigns note the paucity of research evaluating the effectiveness of such strategies (Campbell & Mangenello, this volume). Community education and media campaigns are designed to change people's behavior, either by providing new knowledge or by changing attitudes, but the findings regarding resulting behavior change are inconclusive. There is only slight support for the assumption that a tailored media campaign changes attitudes or affects behavior. In fact, when changes do occur, positive findings are fairly minimal. In a controlled study, Synder (2001) found that only 7% to 10% of those involved in a community campaign changed their behavior. Successful interventions require additional components that actually lead to behavior change (Campbell & Mangenello, 2006).

O'Leary et al. (this volume) recommend a hierarchical system of IPV prevention, depicted as a pyramid. The model's base is a universal prevention program for all individuals, consisting of psychoeducational programs that provide information about norms of behavior within romantic relationships, paired with an active or interactive learning component. Each additional level of the pyramid represents an increasingly intense level of intervention based on the level of physical aggression present. As one moves up the pyramid, interventions become more targeted and focused; different levels of intervention are provided for different levels of the problem.

EMERGING COMMUNITY-BASED APPROACHES TO PREVENTION

The increased study of community over the past decade, and the articulation of strong theoretical models of community capacity, is leading to new prevention approaches. We are moving from observing a "loss of community" to understanding the factors that are related, both positively and negatively, to building community capacity and achieving community outcomes. This understanding has led to the development of strategies and specific activities directed at impacting capacity and outcomes. For example, Bowen, Martin, and Nelson (2002) describe a large-scale community capacity initiative directed at IPV in the military—an initiative that addresses changing the social environment of a group of individuals, rather than attempting to change the individuals directly.

Though individuals perpetrate violence, IPV occurs in community and neighborhood contexts; thus, solutions must focus not only on the individual, but also on the broader environment. The boundaries of intimate relationships are permeable. Since the lives of most people involved in IPV intersect with the broader community, and therefore are subject to community influence, prevention in that larger context can potentially influence what occurs within relationships.

THE NATURE OF COMMUNITIES

Understanding the nature of community, and of a particular community, is a primary consideration in constructing community-level prevention initiatives. Such an understanding clarifies the range of prevention portals and opportunities and informs researchers and program professionals about needed research and possible prevention avenues. Community itself is a potential prevention force and not just a place where prevention activities occur.

Community as a Place: Boundaries of Interest

Boundaries are important because they help to target prevention efforts. Coulton (1995) discusses the phenomenological, interactional, statistical, and political aspects of community boundaries. Phenomenological boundaries are determined by the consensus of people who reside in contiguity; that is, people generally agree that their neighborhood covers a certain land area. An interactional view of community boundaries is concerned with patterns of contact between residents, friends, and acquaintances that occupy the same geographic area. Statistical approaches often employ census information, which provides hard data on the characteristics of occupants of particular land areas. Political boundaries include designations such as towns, districts, counties, wards, and so on.

Sampson (2001) notes the importance of focusing on a spatially oriented conceptualization of community, rather than simply defining community in terms of solidarity among residents. He suggests the neighborhood as a concrete representation of a community. Chaskin et al. (2001) note that when community conceptualization is tied to geography, it includes natural boundaries, a recognized history, and demographic patterns, as well as industries and organizations located in it. They also note that shared social interests and characteristics (e.g., language, customs, class, or ethnicity) can be used to define community. They add that in established communities all of these community elements coalesce to form a unique geographic area inhabited by people with distinct shared characteristics.

Chaskin et al. (2001) and Coulton (1995) note the significance of functional elements of a community. A community attribute may be oriented on the development and delivery of goods and services. As political entities, communities can collectively mobilize around key issues, thereby having another functional element. Communities provide within their boundaries physical spaces and facilities that form the context of social interaction, which may be a visible marker of identity and belonging. Within these boundaries, regardless of how or by whom they are defined, community processes influence people's lives. How we conceptualize the community affects planning research and prevention efforts.

Community as a Prevention Force: Social Organization

Social organization is a significant element in building community capacity (Furstenberg & Hughes, 1997; Mancini, Martin, & Bowen, 2003; Sampson, 2001). Social organization pertains to how people in a community interrelate, cooperate, and provide mutual support, and includes social support norms, social controls that regulate behavior and interaction patterns, and the networks that operate in a community (Furstenberg & Hughes, 1997). Social organizational processes in the community influence individuals within intimate partner relationships. The social organization of individuals, intimate partners, and families within a community provides guidance on structuring and delivering prevention activities.

An important aspect of social organization involves people's expectations of their community life. Sampson (2001) makes an excellent point: "One of the most central of such common goals or ends is the desire of community residents to live in orderly environments free of predatory crime" (p. 8). He defines social organization as "the ability of a community structure to realize the common values of its residents and maintain effective social controls" (p. 8). Social control is important because it is a regulatory mechanism that helps community residents achieve common goals.

Our thinking on social organization is influenced by Furstenberg and Hughes's (1997) work on neighborhood influences on children's well-being. Social relationships exercise powerful and direct influences on individual, relationship, and family well-being; furthermore, those social and intimate partner relationships mediate other community influences. Social capital is both a characteristic and a result of processes reflected in social organization (Putnam, 2000). According to Coleman (1988), the tripartite content of social capital centers on information, reciprocity, and shared norms. Social capital is a facilitating asset for people, an asset that enables them to be more successful in their communities.

Shared norms are of particular interest within the context of preventing IPV since, for instance, the belief that hitting should not be an element of a relationship is an equivocal one (Sabol, Coulton, & Korbin, 2004). For example, Silverman and Williamson (1997) report that between 10% and 25% of males in their sample felt that under certain conditions it is acceptable to abuse women. Furstenberg and Hughes (1997) note that normative support can be provided for both licit and illicit activities; activity considered unacceptable by the general population might be more tolerated among certain subgroups. These subgroups are not necessarily or solely characterized by particular demographic characteristics but also by psychographic characteristics, including attitudes about gender, about sense of self and sense of others, about risk-taking, and so on. Thus, the social organization of a community is a primary prevention portal, whether bound by physical geography, political considerations, or demographic characteristics. Community should be considered as a force in violence prevention rather than only in terms of space and place (Bowen, Gwiasda, & Brown, 2004).

COMMUNITY CAPACITY

Social organization provides an umbrella for the conceptualization of specific group processes and effects that reflect the complexity of community contexts. One such group effect, community capacity, reflects the collective dynamic of a community that comprises and surrounds families (Bowen, Martin, Mancini, & Nelson, 2000). "Building community capacity" represents a conceptual approach to adding an action element to discussions about communities and neighborhoods. Community capacity frameworks are about change and the processes that influence change. The framework assumes that communities can take control of their own destinies, can marshal a range of resources in that regard, and can build a level of community quality and competency that has an ongoing positive influence.

Our community capacity model (see Figure 1) contains four main concepts: (a) community capacity, (b) community results, (c) formal and informal networks, and (d) effect levels (Bowen et al., 2000; Bowen, Martin, Mancini, & Nelson, 2001; Bowen, Mancini, Martin, Ware, & Nelson, 2003; Mancini, Bowen, & Martin, 2005; Mancini et al., 2003). The figure also includes a set of intermediate results that specify the path through which community capacity operates in achieving broad-based community results. Community capacity, the central element of the model, is defined here as

> the degree to which people in a community demonstrate a sense of shared responsibility for the general welfare of the community and its individual members, and also demonstrate collective competence by taking advantage of opportunities for addressing community needs and confronting situations that threaten the safety and well-being of community members. (Bowen et al., 2000, p. 7)

This approach suggests that community capacity is evident in degrees (rather than simply being present or absent), that concern is expressed both for the community in general and for particular parts of the community, that action is taken (rather than just expressions of sentiment), that this action seizes opportunities, and that action occurs with regard to normative, everyday life situations as well as situations that are extraordinary threats.

A key term is *demonstrate* because community capacity includes taking action evidenced by observable results. Community capacity mediates between social capital accruing from formal and informal networks and the achievement of desired community results. Social capital is integral to our model and is the aggregate of resources (including information, opportunities, and instrumental support) that arise from reciprocal social networks and relationships, and that result from participation in formal and informal settings (Coleman, 1988; Putnam, 2000; Sabol et al., 2004). Social capital involves reciprocity and trust among people and is evident in civic engagement, religious groups, member- ship groups, and community initiatives.

FIGURE 1. Community Capacity Approach to Preventing Intimate Partner Violence

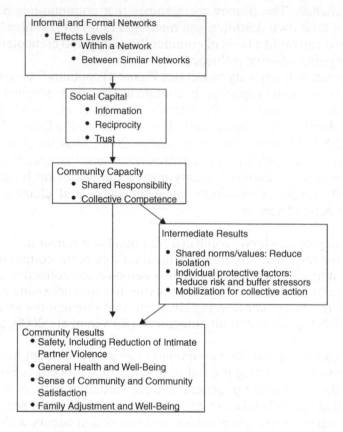

Community Results

Community capacity ultimately leads to community results because it is the demonstration of shared responsibility and of collective competence. Community results are the broad-based, shared outcomes of community members, such as health and well-being (Mancini et al., 2003), safety (Sampson, Raudenbush, & Earls, 1997), and family adaptation (Bowen et al., 2003). *Intermediate community results* identify the specific manner and mechanisms by which community capacity operates to achieve overall community results. As such, intermediate results help structure and guide interventions and provide important markers for evaluation efforts.

Results that are recognized and endorsed by a community provide direction for the targeted use of resources to resolve issues and address concerns. Managing results rather than managing disconnected activities enables efforts to be more intentional, leads to more specific indicators of the success of community efforts, and leads toward discovery about which efforts make an important and desired difference (Orthner & Bowen, 2004). Desired community results are significant because they provide meaning for community capacity, and they are achieved because of community capacity. A focus on community results makes the model more than merely a way to describe community activities. In the current discussion, a community result is the reduction of IPV.

Networks

Formal and informal networks of social care both are vehicles for building community capacity. The former are networks associated with agencies and organizations, whereas the latter are natural networks of relationships with work colleagues, friends, neighbors, and other voluntary relationships (Budde & Schene, 2004). Within each of these networks there is interaction between individuals, but in formal networks the element of obligation is evident. The formal network is usually not the first choice of people in need, whereas people often seek support from informal associations (Beggs, Haines, & Hurlbert, 1996). When these informal systems are not available or are deemed ineffective, then attention turns to formal systems.

Our approach focuses on informal support because it seems to be the preferred source of social care and because we believe it remains a largely untapped source for building healthy communities. Communities, agencies, and organizations are not usually intentional in building informal support networks, yet formal networks can better meet their goals of supporting individuals, families, and communities by mobilizing and empowering the informal network. This approach places emphasis on people and on the community itself, thereby placing a premium on informal networks in the community.

Wills and Shiner (2000) describe five general informal network support functions: (a) emotional support, (b) instrumental support, (c) informational support, (d) companionship, and (e) validation. Emotional support is what we might receive from a confidant, and it often demonstrates caring and approval oriented toward reassuring self-worth; this can motivate people to deal with difficulties they are facing and to believe they can be successful. Instrumental support is tangible and includes provision of money, household assistance, and the like. It is oriented toward solving practical, everyday life problems, and can provide respite for people experiencing stress and difficulties. Informational support is geared toward problem solving, provides information about resources and opportunities, and enhances people's knowledge about methods to resolve issues they are facing. Companionship support is time spent with others and is a socialization mechanism; it provides respite from everyday life demands in that it often includes activities involving sports, outdoor activities, movies and theatre, and trips. Companionship support can create a context for others kinds of support. Finally, validation helps a person understand her or his position in relation to other people facing similar circumstances and concerns. This is particularly important because of the despair that occurs when one feels that a situation is both unusual and insurmountable. Feedback is an important part of validation.

It is evident that the functions potentially found within the informal network of social care are not mutually exclusive; rather, they go hand-in-hand in contributing to well-being. These support functions represent how people establish and maintain intimate partner connections and they reflect the core of social organization.

Effect Levels

The final component of our model is the *effect levels* that describe the operations of formal and informal networks (Small & Supple, 2001). As formal and informal networks operate, several kinds of effects and associations occur. First-level effects occur within a homogeneous network, such as a community mental health center or a neighborhood. Efforts to address an important issue or problem are contained within the network, such as among agency staff working to address increased incidences of partner violence, or among neighbors trying to find ways to support a resident they believe to be a victim of partner violence. In the case of first-level effects, community capacity is increased because members of a single network are bonding around an important community issue (Putnam, 2000).

Second-level effects describe what happens between similar networks, such as between several community agencies dealing with partner violence. In this instance, the focus would be on how professionals from these agencies collaborate and pool their resources to meet a community result of safety in intimate relationships. As applied to the informal network, there may be a number of contiguous neighborhoods banding together to support victims of partner violence, and to share information on improving neighborhood conditions that affect networking or interaction among neighbors.

According to Small and Supple (2001), third-level effects involve interaction between dissimilar networks. An example would be partnerships between community agencies and neighborhood groups for the purpose of providing support for violence victims and for intervening in communities that seem to present a risk of partner violence. These third-level effects are consonant with Putnam's (2000) discussion of bridging. In this case, there is intermingling of formal and informal networks–and the vitality and expertise that accompanies them–to build community capacity and to achieve desired community results (Sabol et al., 2004).

These third-level effects hold the most promise for making a difference in community life because they reflect a more comprehensive, multiple sector approach to IPV. They also elevate the informal network to a position of principal importance, which is consistent with Kretzmann and McKnight's (1993) perspective on building vital communities. For deep and enduring change to occur in communities, community members themselves must be integrally involved in the change process, and there must be a focus on the community's assets rather than solely seeing a community in terms of its problems and deficits.

Community capacity as an aspect of social organization enables researchers to capture the process of community influence on individuals and their relationships. This perspective reveals how informal networks of friends, neighbors, and associates interact; how formal networks of agencies, organizations, and civic groups interact with people and their relationships; and how the interplay of formal and informal networks shapes the relationship between intimate partners. The perspective also allows identification of the actions (reciprocity) and sentiments (trust) in intimate relationships that result from network involvement. Reciprocity and trust lead toward the action dimension (collective competence) and the sentiment dimension (sense of shared responsibility) of community capacity. Community capacity positions individuals to achieve important results for themselves and for their communities.

AIR FORCE SUICIDE PREVENTION PROGRAM:
A COMMUNITY CAPACITY APPROACH

Thus far we have provided a theoretical community capacity framework. A published evaluation of a community capacity approach to the prevention of IPV could not be located. However, one recent evaluation does describe how such an approach has functioned in the prevention of a similar broad-based social problem, suicide, and generalizes to the subject of IPV prevention.

In 1996, the U.S. Air Force instituted a broad-based suicide prevention program based on eleven initiatives in three broad areas: (a) changing the policies and culture of the Air Force to encourage and support help-seeking behavior; (b) reengineering the Air Force human service system to provide better service to clients through collaboration and partnerships; and (c) providing a comprehensive, four-tiered system of suicide prevention and awareness training to all members of the community.

The overarching thrust of these initiatives was to change the norms and culture of the Air Force and in particular to remove the stigma associated with asking for help. Essentially, the Air Force focused on creating a network of social care. A fundamental objective of the program was to change overall community behavior, with the smallest work units becoming the locus for change. Specifically, work units were educated on suicide awareness and prevention within a "buddy-care" context: each member of a work unit was to note the status of his or her immediate co-worker, to pay attention to that co-worker's mood, and to provide support if needed. Thus, a key target of change was the sense of shared responsibility and collective competence among work units.

During the first year following implementation of the suicide prevention program, the number of suicides in the Air Force dropped 80%. Since that time, the Air Force has maintained a significant reduction in suicide rates as well as reductions in other social problem behaviors, including IPV. An independent external evaluation (Knox, Litts, Talcott, Feig, & Caine, 2003), while cautious about attributing causality, ruled out potential confounding factors as explanations for the decline. It also identified expected changes in measurable desired intermediate outcomes, such as decreased rates of homicide, accidental death, violent offenses, and lessened severity of family violence.

What was operating here and what is its relevance, if any, to prevention of IPV? First, the state of suicide prevention research, as reflected in the literature, is very similar to the state of IPV research. There are few empirical studies; there is a focus on individual behavior; and there is a reactive approach that favors targeting sites where individuals with suicidal ideation may appear, such as mental health crisis services, hotlines, or emergency room and other medical facilities. The only community-level intervention consists of media and public awareness campaigns.

The Air Force results have been attributed to a number of factors directly relevant and applicable to the development of community-based IPV prevention efforts. These factors include the program's framework, process, and approach, as well as its specific intervention strategies. The organizational and structural aspects of the program are key to its success. First, the Air Force adopted as its starting point the Centers for Disease Control and Prevention's (1992, 1999) consensus recommendations for population-based prevention approaches. This ensured its program would be grounded in strong science by using a rigorous data-driven prevention planning model to guide its analysis and understanding of the problem and associated issues. The program's 11 initiatives were the result of this process.

The IPV literature acknowledges the importance of community. However, coordinated community response efforts typically have been limited to a single segment of the community–the criminal justice community. In contrast, the Air Force suicide prevention program adopted a broad-based total community approach with strong leadership support. While suicide traditionally has been considered a medical issue, the Air Force program was not a traditional stovepipe response. Rather, a community-wide, cross-functional team developed it with representatives from all Air Force constituencies, including community members. Second, key intervention strategies focused on modifying community behavior and on developing collective efficacy of work units. Finally, the program adopted an absolute requirement for collaboration and partnerships among the Air Force's formal helping agencies. The Air Force model presents community as the organizing concept in its planning and development, in its prevention strategies, and in its program execution.

IMPLICATIONS FOR PROGRAM DEVELOPMENT

Current prevention practices directed at reducing the prevalence of IPV are limited predominately to media campaigns, public service announcements, and universal dating violence prevention education classes. Most often these programs are directed at changing behaviors and social norms. These are critical outcomes, but as the research data shows, these interventions have been mostly ineffective in changing either behavior or norms, mainly due to their limited scope, individual focus, and one-time or short-term nature. Coordinated community response practices have brought about impressive changes over the past decade, including mobilizing the criminal justice system to be more responsive to victims and to hold offenders accountable. However, they have not brought about the desired changes in reduction of IPV.

Our review suggests several paths for future program development. First, it is critical to move beyond isolated program efforts and to begin designing comprehensive, multilevel, community-based strategies for the prevention of IPV. Redundancy and mutual reinforcement are critical to broad-based change.

Second, the focus on individuals and on individual-level changes in attitudes and behavior must expand to include a broad focus on the norms and social context in which the behavior occurs. Targeting social norms directly enhances the reciprocal nature between norms and individual behavior. Reflecting the widespread renewal of attention to community, Levine (1998) makes a persuasive case that an orientation on the individual is no longer sufficient for prevention planning. He argues that prevention efforts designed from an ecological perspective can change norms and result in more a positive social climate.

Third, in the language of our community capacity model, current interventions focus almost exclusively on changes within formal agencies and systems for intervening in IPV, with little or no attention given to the potential of informal networks. This represents a missed opportunity, especially in light of the knowledge that most individuals-in-need turn to informal supports rather than formal agencies. McKnight (1995) identifies the risks of relying on formal agencies, suggesting that doing so supplants the capacity of informal networks and associations. There is untapped potential capacity in individuals' informal networks, associations, and communities. Prevention programs intentionally designed to tap that capacity in the service of reduction of IPV can pay impressive dividends.

Thus, a new comprehensive approach is required in order to improve IPV prevention efforts. We recommend expanding the emerging framework described by O'Leary et al. (this volume). The O'Leary et al. model has the potential to function as an organizing framework to structure IPV prevention and intervention efforts. It provides a comprehensive, targeted, and tailored approach to resource allocation.

We propose a new base for the O'Leary et al. pyramid (this volume), one that employs community as an organizing concept. Embracing community as an organizing concept acknowledges that from a systems or ecological perspective community represents a primary focus of prevention efforts. Community as an organizing concept is operationalized in three ways: (a) community as a place for prevention, (b) community as a target of intervention, and (c) community as a force for intervention.

Community as a Place for Prevention

Any prevention effort needs to account for community boundaries because these boundaries identify both resources–agencies, organizations, churches, and close-knit groups–and deficits. Accounting for a breadth of definitions of community allows for development of a roadmap of the community elements available to program professionals. An ecology of the community thus emerges that identifies the various layers of community and shows the sources of influence on people in a community, such as physical space and facilities, agency and organization locations, and so on.

Community as a Target for Prevention

In addition to directly targeting community norms, the community-capacity approach focuses directly on the development of informal social care networks to enhance capacity and to obtain positive results. Through networks of connections and social care, community capacity emerges and produces three key intermediate outcomes: (a) incorporation of shared norms and values inconsistent with interpersonal violence; (b) enhancement of individual protective factors, which reduces the probability of IPV and buffers the impact of such violence; and (c) the development of community skills, resources, and competence to engage in collective community action (i.e., to intervene in IPV). These outcomes represent the mechanisms thorough which community capacity accomplishes a reduction of IPV.

Community as a Force for Prevention

The ultimate aim of a community-capacity approach is to facilitate the mobilization of community members–to empower their direct involvement and sense of ownership–toward the articulation, development, and implementation of resident-led comprehensive strategies that yield positive results in the face of challenges and opportunities. When this occurs, community has become a powerful force in the lives of its citizens.

Our review of the Air Force suicide prevention program suggests that at least three additional elements are necessary for a successful community-capacity approach to IPV prevention. These elements include (a) a team of leaders who share a sense of ownership and vision, (b) community engagement in the development of a strategic plan, and (c) an infrastructure to support program delivery. Notably, these elements do not include specific prevention programs.

We suggest that the range of existing programs, including media campaigns, psychoeducational programs, and coordinated community responses, should remain a part of the comprehensive set of prevention activities. What is different is that the community-capacity approach embeds these elements within a larger contextual framework that demands a comprehensive focus across multiple facets of the community, specifically centering on building connections and empowering informal networks to develop and mobilize newfound community capacity in the service of community- and resident-identified initiatives and outcomes.

IMPLICATIONS FOR RESEARCH

There appear to be relatively few studies that connect community dimensions with IPV, though research connecting community and prevention is emergent. Few studies focus on IPV and community factors, but there are studies demonstrating connections between community factors and child maltreatment (Garbarino & Kostelny, 1992) and other forms of violence (Sampson et al., 1997).

However, two recent empirical studies do address IPV issues, to a limited extent. Miles-Doan (1998) analyzed one Florida county's law enforcement data and found higher rates of IPV in neighborhoods with higher measures of social disadvantage, such as greater poverty, more unemployed males, and more female-headed households with young children. She notes that the significance of neighborhood effects for explaining IPV is less than the significance of those effects for explaining violence among other acquaintances. Nevertheless, while discussing steps to improve models of IPV, Miles-Doan points to the importance of some aspects of social organization and community capacity (e.g., community members' perceptions that violence is a problem, and residents' willingness to intervene in a intimate partner dispute).

A second relevant study is an empirical analysis of Canadian quality-of-life survey data (Dekeseredy, Schwartz, Alvi, & Tomaszewski, 2003). These researchers examine the relationship between perceived collective efficacy (i.e., a sense of shared responsibility and collective competence) and women's victimization in public housing neighborhoods. Though the statistical relationship is only weakly significant, respondents lower in collective efficacy are more likely to identify themselves as victims of IPV. Dekeseredy et al. note that their data suggest community antiviolence programs have little effect on violence against women within intimate relationships. This research is significant in that it suggests that collective efficacy, which parallels community capacity, holds promise for understanding community effects on IPV.

Community Layers

Definitions of community are important for program professionals and researchers alike, who must consider boundaries when enacting prevention initiatives. Of particular importance to the research component of IPV prevention is what definitions of community suggest about the layers of community life. Each layer is a component of the community that can be examined and that represents an intervention portal. For example, a geographic view of community attends to the juxtaposition of where people live, where they procure goods and services, and where formal network support is located. A geographic view also includes where people congregate and the density of their living arrangements. A comprehensive research approach to preventive influences and effects would account for these aspects of community geography, which may influence people's engagement in the community and in prevention activities.

A second community definition might consider statistical parameters. Census-like data may indicate pockets of greater rates of violence in general, of child maltreatment, or of IPV. If these data are available, then they should be accounted for in research planning, especially in the case of research designed to capture program effects. It can be misleading to study a phenomenon that is either over- or underrepresented within a community. Thus, depending on what researchers and program professionals want to know, it may be desirable to focus on areas where there are greater or lesser rates of violence (or other community characteristics, for that matter).

Network Types and Their Nexus

From a practice perspective, knowing which aspects of community influence IPV levels enables more informed program development and evaluation. The community capacity literature discusses informal and formal networks and their nexus. What is not known is the relative influence of these networks on quality of life–whether that quality is measured by how well people like where they live or is measured by the use of violence as a way to resolve problems and vent frustrations. Consequently, a primary research question has to focus on teasing apart elements of community life and examining their role in either mitigating or exacerbating IPV.

More particularly, and of great significance in the community capacity model, is the necessity for a close examination of the relationships between informal and formal networks of social care (Budde & Schene, 2004). Important research issues include how formal networks engage informal networks in prevention activities, how the informal network supports formal networks and contributes to their viability, and whether each of these networks of social care is functioning in the most appropriate, efficient, and successful ways. We subscribe to the opinion that formal networks should not replace informal networks; that is, formal networks should not deny informal systems their rightful and preferred place of influence in people's lives. However, we also believe that formal networks play an important role in communities: to support well-functioning informal networks, and in the case of IPV, to provide support that informal networks may be unprepared to provide.

Explanatory Models of IPV

Another primary research question is how community elements compare with other factors in explaining, understanding, and predicting IPV (Guterman, 2004). Because so little research has been conducted in this area, it is difficult to know if the findings are artifacts of conceptualization and measurement or if they truly reflect the relevance of community factors. There certainly may be individual or family factors that act as the primary determinants of IPV; however, community factors including social disadvantage may influence those individual and family factors (Sabol et al., 2004). Even if community elements are relatively less significant for explaining the incidence of IPV, it may still be important from a prevention perspective to understand how they might be used to promote more positive relationships within communities.

Need for Comparative Studies

The community capacity model defines community capacity as sense of shared responsibility and collective competence, and suggests that when these elements are stronger there are positive results for communities. However, we assume that people within informal networks also possess these characteristics and that they will act in certain ways because they are high in capacity. But does this hold with regard to a severe social problem such as IPV? To what degree is there community capacity among friends and neighbors when IPV is the issue? Do they feel a sense of shared responsibility in the case of IPV, and do they exhibit that tendency to collectively make a positive difference? In a broader sense, what indications are there that a community will address tough social problems such as IPV? These are primary questions for research, which in turn will have important implications for program development.

One research approach that may have merit in understanding how community connections permeate couples' lives, and the positive or negative influence of these connections, is to examine extreme groups. For example, what is the nature of community connections among couples that are violence-free? In contrast, what is the nature of the informal network of social care among those who are violent? There may be marked differences in the two groups' friend and neighbor networks, in their associations with confidants outside of the couple relationship, or in the value placed on these connections. There may also be differences in the values, qualities, and behaviors of the two groups, or in the people who comprise the informal network of friends, neighbors, and other associates.

The content of what transpires within the informal network may also differ. For example, our earlier discussion of types of social support demonstrates that support is far-ranging, includes instrumental and affective elements, and can function in identity formation. An interesting research question is, what kind of social support exercises more relative impact on a person's behavior and values? A related applied research question is, which aspects of social support can be mobilized to prevent IPV? An underlying assumption is that informal networks do have an impact on adult behaviors, attitudes, and values.

Evaluation Research

As community-capacity-oriented prevention programs are developed and implemented, an equally important corollary is evaluation (Guterman, 2004; Mancini, Huebner, McCollum, & Marek, 2005). Overall, IPV preventions are not known for rigorous evaluation of program effects, either formative or summative. But unless programs are systematically evaluated and accordingly adjusted, they remain intentions-based rather than science-based. A particular research avenue is to examine how coordinated community responses affect IPV. The community capacity model places importance on collaboration and partnerships (see Figure 1, Effects Levels), yet there is little empirical evidence about how such collaborations would enhance IPV prevention. There is a more nuanced question as well: What combination of formal network members (agencies and organizations) provides the more effective approach to IPV prevention? A primary evaluation science question is *what* works for *whom*, and *when* does it work? In order to demonstrate how a community capacity approach influences reduction in IPV, researchers need to be specific about measuring their desired results (this involves identifying a reasonable target rate), clearly defining and measuring community components (an example being elements of informal networks), monitoring the intensity of a community-oriented prevention effort (this raises the issue of dosage and exposure), and determining an informed timeline on when results should be evident (this requires a strong formative and summative evaluation approach).

CONCLUSION

We assume that the prevention of IPV largely depends on both informal and formal network connections within communities. Community capacity ultimately resides with people in the community because it is their sense of shared responsibility and collective competence, marshaled to bring about the conditions they desire, that make positive differences in their lives. How intimate partners interact and how they solve disagreements and problems are amenable to influence by community networks, if those networks are wise to the problems and are equally wise to the solutions. A community capacity approach is multilayered and recognizes that change emerges from resilient community members and from viable institutions in the community, and from the partnerships they develop to prevent IPV.

REFERENCES

Bachman, R. (1994). *National crime victimization report: Violence against women.* Washington, DC: U.S. Department of Justice.

Beggs, J. J., Haines, V. A., & Hurlbert, J. S. (1996). Situational contingencies surrounding the receipt of informal support. *Social Forces, 75*, 201-222.

Bowen, G. L., Mancini, J. A., Martin, J. A., Ware, W. B., & Nelson, J. P. (2003). Promoting the adaptation of military families: An empirical test of a community practice model. *Family Relations: Interdisciplinary Journal of Applied Family Studies, 52*, 33-44.

Bowen, G. L., Martin, J. A., & Nelson, J. P. (2002) A community capacity response to family violence in the military. In A. R. Roberts & G. J. Greene (Eds.), *Social workers' desk reference* (pp. 551-556). New York: Oxford Press.

Bowen, G. L., Martin, J. A., Mancini, J. A., & Nelson, J. P. (2000). Community capacity: Antecedents and consequences. *Journal of Community Practice, 8*, 1-21.

Bowen, G. L., Martin, J. A., Mancini, J. A., & Nelson, J. P. (2001). Civic engagement and sense of community in the military. *Journal of Community Practice, 9*, 71-93.

Bowen, L. K., Gwiasda, V., & Brown, M. M. (2004). Engaging community residents to prevent violence. *Journal of Interpersonal Violence, 19*, 356-367.

Budde, S., & Schene, P. (2004). Informal social support interventions and their role in violence prevention. *Journal of Interpersonal Violence, 19*, 341-355.

Campbell, J. C., & Manganello, J. (2006). Changing public attitudes as a prevention strategy to reduce intimate partner violence. *Journal of Aggression, Maltreatment & Trauma, 13*(3/4), 13-39.

Centers for Disease Control and Prevention. (1992). *Youth suicide prevention programs: A resource guide.* Atlanta, GA: US Department of Health and Human Services, Public Health Service.

Centers for Disease Control and Prevention. (1999). Suicide prevention among active duty Air Force personnel, United States, 1990-1999. *Morbidity and Mortality Weekly Report, 48*, 1053-1057.

Chaskin, R. J., Brown, P., Venkatesh, S., & Vidal, A. (2001). *Building community capacity.* New York: Aldine De Gruyter.

Coleman, J. (1988). Social capital in the creation of human capital. *American Journal of Sociology, 94*, S95-S120.

Coulton, C. J. (1995). Using community-level indicators of children's well-being in comprehensive community initiatives. In J. P. Connell, A. C. Kubisch, L. B. Schorr, & C. H. Weiss (Eds.), *New approaches to evaluating community initiatives: Concepts, methods, and contexts* (pp. 173-199). Washington, DC: The Aspen Institute.

Daro, D., Edleson, J. L., & Pinderhughes, H. (2004). Finding common ground in the study of child maltreatment, youth violence, and adult domestic violence. *Journal of Interpersonal Violence, 19*, 282-298.

Dekeseredy, W. S., Schwartz, M. D., Alvi, S., & Tomaszewski, E. A. (2003). Perceived collective efficacy and women's victimization in public housing. *Criminal Justice, 3*, 5-27.

Department of Justice. (1984). *Report of the Attorney General's Task Force on Family Violence.* Washington, DC: U.S. Department of Justice.

Feld, S. L., & Straus, M. A. (1989). Escalation and resistance of wife assault in marriage. *Criminology, 27,* 141-161.

Furstenberg, F. F., & Hughes, M. E. (1997). The influence of neighborhoods on children's development: A theoretical perspective and a research agenda. In J. Brooks-Gunn, G. J. Duncan, & J. L. Aber (Eds.), *Neighborhood poverty (Vol. 2): Policy implications in studying neighborhoods* (pp. 23-47). New York: Russell Sage Foundation.

Garbarino, J. & Kostelny, K., (1992). Child maltreatment as a community problem. *Child Abuse and Neglect, 16,* 455-464.

Guterman, N. B. (2004). Advancing prevention research on child abuse, youth violence, and domestic violence: Emerging strategies and issues. *Journal of Interpersonal Violence, 19,* 299-321.

Jones, A. A., Gielen, A. C., Campbell, J. C., Schollenberger, J., Dienemann, J. A., Kub, J. et al. (1999). Annual and lifetime prevalence of partner abuse in a sample of female HMO enrollees. *Women's Health Issues, 9,* 295-305.

Knox, K. L., Litts, D. A., Talcott, G. W., Feig, J. C., & Caine, E. D. (2003). Risk of suicide and related adverse outcomes after exposure to a suicide prevention programme in the US Air Force: Cohort study. *British Medical Journal, 327,* 1376-1380.

Kretzmann, J. P., & McKnight, J. L. (1993). *Building communities from the inside out: A path toward finding and mobilizing a community's assets.* Chicago: Acta Publications.

Levine, M. (1998). Prevention and community. *American Journal of Community Psychology, 26,* 189-206.

Mancini, J. A., Bowen, G. L., & Martin, J. A. (2005). Families in community contexts. In V. Bengtson, A. Acock, K. Allen, & P. Dilworth-Anderson (Eds.), *Sourcebook of family theory and research* (pp. 293-306). Beverly Hills, CA: Sage.

Mancini, J. A., Huebner, A. J., McCollum, E., & Marek, L. I. (2005). Evaluation science and family therapy. In D. Sprenkle & F. P. Piercy (Eds.), *Research methods in family therapy* (pp. 272-296). New York: Praeger.

Mancini, J. A., Martin, J. A., & Bowen, G. L. (2003). Community capacity. In T. P. Gullotta & M. Bloom (Eds.), *Encyclopedia of primary prevention and health promotion* (pp. 319-330). New York: Kluwer Academic/Plenum.

McKnight, J. (1995). *The careless society: Community and its counterfeits.* New York: Basic Books.

Miles-Doan, R. (1998). Violence between spouses and intimates: Does neighborhood context matter? *Social Forces, 77,* 623-638.

National Violence Against Women Prevention Research Center. (2002). *Violence against women prevention programming: Report of what is in use.* Retrieved November 30, 2003 from the National Violence Against Women Prevention Research Center website, http://www.vawprevention.2006/

O'Leary, K. D., Woodin, E. M., & Fritz, P. T. (2006). Prevention of aggression in intimate partner relationships. *Journal of Aggression, Maltreatment & Trauma, 13*(3/4), 121-178.

Orthner, D. K., & Bowen, G. L. (2004). Strengthening practice through results management. In A. R. Roberts, & K. Yeager (Eds.), *Handbook of practice based research* (pp. 897-904). New York: Oxford University Press.

Pence, E. (1983). The Duluth domestic abuse intervention project. *Hamline Law Review, 6,* 247-275.

Putnam, R. D. (2000). *Bowling alone*. New York: Simon & Schuster.

Rennison, C. M. (2003). *Intimate partner violence, 1993-2001*. Washington, DC: U.S. Department of Justice.

Sabol, W. J., Coulton, C. J., & Korbin, J. E. (2004). Building community capacity for violence prevention. *Journal of Interpersonal Violence, 19*, 322-340.

Sampson, R. J. (2001). How do communities undergird or undermine human development? Relevant contexts and social mechanisms. In A. Booth & A. C. Crouter (Eds.), *Does it take a village? Community effects on children, adolescents, and families* (pp. 3-30). Mahwah, NJ: Erlbaum.

Sampson, R. J., Raudenbush, S. W., & Earls, F. (1997). Neighborhoods and violent crime: A multilevel study of collective efficacy. *Science, 277*, 918-924.

Shepard, M. (1999). *Evaluation coordinated community responses to domestic violence*. Retrieved January 28, 2003 from the Violence Against Women Online Resources Website, http://www.vaw.umn.edu/documents/vawnet/ccr/ccr.html#top

Silverman, J. G., & Williamson, G. M. (1997). Social ecology and entitlements involved in battering by heterosexual college males: Contributions of family and peers. *Violence and Victims, 12*, 147-164.

Small, S., & Supple, A. (2001). Communities as systems: Is a community more than the sum of its parts? In A. Booth & A.C. Crouter (Eds.), *Does it take a village? Community effects on children, adolescents, and families* (pp. 161-174). Mahwah, NJ: Erlbaum.

Snyder, L. B. (2001). How effective are mediated health campaigns? In R. E. Rice & C. K. Atkin (Eds.), *Public communication campaigns* (pp. 181-192). Thousand Oaks, CA: Sage.

Tjaden, P., & Thoennes, N. (2000). Prevalence and consequences of male to female and female-to-male intimate partner violence as measured by the National Violence Against Women Survey. *Violence Against Women, 6*, 142-161.

Wills, T. A., & Shiner, O. (2000). Measuring perceived and received social support. In S. Cohen, L. G. Underwood, & B. H. Gottlieb (Eds.), *Social support measurement and intervention* (pp. 86-135). New York: Oxford.

Wolfe, D. A., & Jaffe, P. G. (2003). *Prevention of domestic violence and sexual assault*. Retrieved November 24, 2003 from the Violence Against Women Online Resources Website, http://www.vaw.umn.edu/documents/vawnet/arprevent/arprevent.html

doi:10.1300/J146v13n03_08

CONCLUSION

Future Directions in Intimate Partner Violence Prevention Research

Sandra M. Stith, PhD

SUMMARY. During the past 20 years, research on dynamics of intimate partner violence, risk factors, and treatment of intimate partner violence has flourished. However, research on the prevention of intimate partner violence is in its infancy. The current volume was developed in order to examine the state of the art in preventing intimate partner violence. To that end, this article offers a synthesis of recommendations for future research made by the authors in this volume and participants in the symposium on the prevention of intimate partner violence sponsored by the Department of Defense. A goal in compiling these recommendations is to foster more and better research into preventing intimate partner violence. doi:10.1300/J146v13n03_09 *[Article copies available for a fee from The Haworth Document Delivery Service: 1-800-HAWORTH. E-mail address:*

Address correspondence to: Sandra M. Stith, PhD, 7054 Haycock Road, Falls Church, VA 22043 (E-mail: sstith@vt.edu).

[Haworth co-indexing entry note]: "Future Directions in Intimate Partner Violence Prevention Research." Stith, Sandra M. Co-published simultaneously in *Journal of Aggression, Maltreatment & Trauma* (The Haworth Maltreatment & Trauma Press, an imprint of The Haworth Press, Inc.) Vol. 13, No. 3/4, 2006, pp. 229-244; and: *Prevention of Intimate Partner Violence* (ed: Sandra M. Stith) The Haworth Maltreatment & Trauma Press, an imprint of The Haworth Press, Inc., 2006, pp. 229-244. Single or multiple copies of this article are available for a fee from The Haworth Document Delivery Service [1-800-HAWORTH, 9:00 a.m. - 5:00 p.m. (EST). E-mail address: docdelivery@haworthpress.com].

KEYWORDS. Intimate partner violence, prevention, future research, health care screening, media, prevention programming

One goal of this book is to foster more and better research into preventing intimate partner violence (IPV). Each of the preceding manuscripts has made it clear that IPV has serious long-term impact on individuals, families, and society in general. In addition, each of the authors has reviewed the state-of the art in research and offered implications for individuals who work to prevent IPV and suggestions for future research. In this manuscript, these ideas will be summarized, along with some of the ideas developed by working groups of researchers who participated in the Department of Defense (DOD) sponsored symposium on the prevention of IPV.

In 1988, David Finkelhor, Gerald Hotaling, and Kersti Yllo published a book, *Stopping Family Violence: Research Priorities in the Coming Decade*. In this book, the authors invited some of the leading domestic violence researchers, practitioners, and activists to think of research projects that would be of importance to stopping family violence. These experts developed one proposal in the area of spouse abuse prevention. The study they proposed was designed to "evaluate the effectiveness of a variety of approaches to spouse abuse prevention" and "to contrast various modes of presenting spouse abuse education materials to students" (p. 91). They proposed that the study be longitudinal (from 6 to 10 years). They wanted to randomly assign a variety of prevention programs to a large group of students aged 10 to 17, and planned to assess the impact of the prevention program in both the short and long term. In the short term, they wanted to see if the concepts were learned and retained. In the long term, they wanted to see if the students receiving the preventive programs were less likely to be involved in violent dating or marital relationships. Sixteen years later, this study has still not been conducted and we still do not have any data about the real effectiveness of dating violence prevention programming in the schools. It is our hope that research proposals generated at the Department of Defense Symposium and contributed by the authors in this volume will not wait sixteen years to be conducted.

RESEARCH PROPOSALS DEVELOPED AT DOD SYMPOSIUM

Participants at the Department of Defense-supported symposium on prevention of IPV came up with recommendations for future IPV prevention research. Participants at the symposium were divided into three groups: Public Awareness Group, Health Care Screening Group, and Prevention Programming Group. A list of participants in each group is included in the Appendix to this article. Each working group developed a number of proposals. The entire group of participants rank-ordered the entire group of proposals. The highest priority proposals from each working group are included here. In addition, the lower priority research proposals and/or questions from each working group are summarized here. While most of these proposals target active duty service members and their families, these same studies could be adapted to civilian communities.

HIGH PRIORITY RESEARCH PROPOSALS

Public Awareness Group

Working title: "A Call to Action" or "Coaching Boys into Men:" Evaluation of a Public Education Campaign Directed toward Engaging Men in Preventing IPV.

Rationale

The rationale of this study is to address the need to engage men in preventing IPV. Prior U.S. general population surveys have shown men to be less involved and concerned than women about IPV. Even so, the majority of men are concerned and willing to take action, but uncertain as to what they can do. Men compose the majority of the military and majority of IPV perpetrators, but past IPV campaigns have usually "indicted; not invited" men.

Goals

1. To formulate a research-based public education campaign to prevent IPV.
2. To engage men in promoting nonviolence and preventing IPV.

3. To change the social norms tolerating violence against women and girls.
4. To teach boys and young men that violence against women is wrong.
5. To evaluate the effectiveness of the public education campaign.

Description

Recently, a national survey of a civilian population of men asked what IPV prevention activity they were willing to do. The largest group chose teaching their sons and other young boys in their lives that violence against women and girls was wrong. The Family Violence Prevention Fund and Advertiser Council developed a public service campaign designed to encourage this behavior.

This project would replicate the same process among military populations and evaluate the effectiveness of a public education campaign promoting the activity many men say they are willing to do. This could not only prevent IPV among young boys, but also help to change the norms about IPV among the men who are doing the teaching.

The project would entail the same kind of population-based survey with the addition of ethnic- and pay grade-specific focus groups among active duty military men and spouses of active duty women. Like the project upon which it is based, the survey will determine what activities men from different segments of the military–different age groups, pay grades, occupational specialties, ethnic and service groups–are willing to do to promote nonviolence and prevent IPV.

Public education campaign media experts would then work with military public affairs and communication experts, IPV experts, and community participants to design the appropriate campaign (including messenger, message and mode of delivery) to promote the nonviolence activity. The campaign would then be implemented and evaluated, using five waves of surveys conducted before, during, and after the campaign, measuring exposure and impact on attitudes and behavior (enactment of the prevention of violence activity).

Target Population

The study population would include active duty men and male military spouses aged 18 to 30 and, indirectly, their sons and the youth in their lives. The sample would be drawn from four target installations (three stateside and one overseas) and four comparison installations.

Data Collection Method

Methods include random sample surveys at workplace for active duty males and telephone surveys for male spouses of active duty women, as well as focus groups.

Design and Analysis (Three Phases)

Phase 1 consists of a random sample, population-based survey administered at the work place, and a telephone survey for civilian spouses. The survey would ask men about their attitudes, knowledge, and behaviors regarding IPV (e.g., how serious a problem is IPV, knowledge of victims or perpetrators, actions to address IPV in the past; if none, why, etc.) and also about what they are willing to do to prevent IPV. Focus groups would also be carried out with analysis by ethnicity, pay grade, and occupational group.

Phase 2 focuses on campaign development, including input from military and civilian public education campaign professionals, IPV experts, military community participants, and military public affairs experts. These professionals would work together to design the campaign message, mode of transmission (print, radio and TV–civilian and military), avenues of transmission (e.g., exercise venues, bars), and messengers. Additionally, messages should be pilot tested in different groups.

Phase 3 encompasses the evaluation. This phase involves successive random sample cross sectional population-based surveys at the work place, and telephone surveys for civilian spouses. There should be two surveys pre-campaign, one during, one 1-2 months post-campaign, one 6 months post-campaign, and one 12 months post-campaign. These surveys would compare respondents on target and control military installations, as well as those exposed versus not exposed. Exposure can be measured by recall of campaign, responses to a content-based recall question, and responses to a query of respondent's mode of exposure (e.g., TV, radio, print).

Sample

Power analysis will be carried out to determine the sample size needed for surveys with effect size of .10. Focus groups would consist of 8 to 10 volunteers per group, with 16 groups. There should be two focus groups per race/ethnicity category and these should be split by officer/enlisted status (e.g., African American, Anglo, Asian-Pacific Islanders, Latino; two officer, two enlisted each).

Length of Research Project

The project is expected to last five years. Year 1 would focus in Internal Review Board (IRB) approval, collaborative team formation, preliminary survey, and focus groups. Year 2 would involve public education campaign and dissemination plan formulation, and as well as piloting. Year 3 through 5 would see the campaign launched and fully evaluated.

Estimated Costs

Costs are estimated at $500,000 per year for a total of $2.5 million. This reflects an estimate of $500,000 for the campaign and $2 million for the evaluation.

Pros

The proposal is exciting, innovative, targets men, is based on prior research, and takes advantage of military demographics and a captive audience for military media. There are no additional expenses for military media air and print time, and there are ready-made comparison communities.

Cons

The project will be expensive to administer and carry out correctly.

Health Care Screening Group

Working Title: A Longitudinal Study of Screening and Intervention in the Medical Setting.

Rationale

This project will evaluate outcomes to women experiencing IPV who receive a targeted IPV intervention with their medical care versus those who receive standard care. No data currently exist to show that identification and intervention in the medical setting is effective in prevention of IPV.

Goals

This project would evaluate the effectiveness of a three-pronged intervention trial in a medical setting.

Brief Description (Three Phases)

Phase I would involve a determination of outcomes to be studied. An expert panel would be convened to determine appropriate outcome measures. These measures potentially include:

1. Level of emotional abuse using Women's Experience of Battering screening.
2. Level of physical violence.
3. Quality of life.
4. Perception of safety compared to safety assessment tool.

Phase 1 would also entail the use of qualitative methodology to evaluate, from current and former IPV victims, the positive outcomes they identify as important, as well as any unintended negative outcomes.

Phase 2 would evaluate the outcomes, as specified during Phase 1, of the following three alternative interventions in a primary care setting:

1. Intervention 1–Screen and refer.
2. Intervention 2–Screen and provide a brief intervention in the office.
3. Intervention 3–Screen and refer to an advocate.

Design

The project would involve longitudinal randomized control trials in multiple centers.

Data Collection Method

Data collection methods include surveys, focus groups, and in-depth interviews.

Sample

The sample would consist of women, both active duty service members and civilian wives of male active duty service members from three installation hospitals, one per each Military Department identified in OB/GYN, Family Medicine, and Primary Care. The sample would include approximately 5,000 women.

Length of Research Project

The length of the project is estimated at five years.

Estimated Costs

The estimated cost is $3.5 million over five years.

Pros

An advantage of this study would be that it involves a "captive" group, in a screening and intervention environment in which many factors can be controlled.

Cons

The primary drawback of the study is predicted to be attrition due to mandatory reporting.

Prevention Programming Group

Working Title: Do Prevention and Intervention Programs that Target Risk Factors for Partner Violence Have Any Effect on Partner Violence?

Rationale

The rationale of this study is to help determine how prevention programs (e.g., parent education, substance abuse, mental health, stress management, communication, financial management) impact IPV or program related goals.

Goals

The study will determine which IPV risk-related prevention programs help decrease partner violence.

Methods

The study will be a quasi-experimental design, employing the following data collection procedures:

1. Pre-test, post-test, and follow-up measures of IPV attitudes and behaviors.
2. Program-related outcome measures, which include a 1- and 2-year follow-up.
3. Self-report, medical, and other records.

Sample

The sample would consist of active duty military members and spouses who complete selected prevention/intervention programs currently being offered. Number required would be 2,000 (i.e., approximately 200 per program).

Length of Project

The length of the study is estimated at three years.

Estimated Costs

Costs for the project will be approximately $500,000.

Pros

This project can be kept at relatively low costs by leveraging existing programs and methodology. The study will provide needed data on the effectiveness of existing programs in preventing domestic violence.

LIST OF ADDITIONAL RESEARCH RECOMMENDATIONS FROM THE DOD SYMPOSIUM

The following is a list of some of the other research recommendations made by the three working groups at the Department of Defense Symposium.

1. A study using a public awareness campaign to promote resiliency for protective behavior to reduce the harm from exposure to IPV in girls and women. The aim is to help girls/women develop protective traits so if exposed to IPV, they may be able to influence the result.

2. A research study to determine the most effective method of investing resources in public education on IPV by formulating an effective public education campaign on domestic violence with the segments of the military population most at risk for domestic violence. This would be a multi-method study involving focus groups, interviews, and surveys.

3. Use the core competencies in IPV established by the Institute of Medicine (IOM) as a framework to develop, test, and evaluate a core curriculum for medical personnel in domestic violence.

4. A longitudinal study to perform analysis of factors related to cessation and escalation of IPV. The goal of this study is to identify rates of IPV and correlates with cessation/escalation of IPV over time.

5. Comparison study of general versus specific prevention program outcomes. Specifically, this research would compare generalized skill building prevention programs with partner violence focused programs.

6. Compare curricula that address protective factors versus risk factors versus both.

7. Evaluate changes in the role of women in the military and other factors affecting aggression by women.

8. Fatality review and use information and statistics to provide feedback to existing IPV prevention programs.

SUGGESTIONS FOR FUTURE RESEARCH BASED ON ARTICLES IN THIS VOLUME

The authors in this volume offered additional valuable suggestions to guide future research on prevention of intimate partner violence. Dr. Hamby reported that while there is similarity in both process and content among most partner violence prevention programs, fundamental questions remain unanswered about these programs. She suggests that we need research to help us know who to target, what to present, when in the life-span to present the information, where to present it, and whether the prevention programs have any long-term effect on preventing IPV. She makes a strong case for the importance of cost-benefit analyses in future research in the area of partner violence prevention. We need to know whether it makes more sense to offer universal or targeted prevention programs. We need to know the costs of universal versus targeted programs and the cost of prevention versus the long-term costs of partner violence. We also need research to help us know whether the partner violence prevention programs should be embedded in general prevention programming or should be offered as distinct curricula. Outcome studies that manipulate the elements of the curricula are needed to identify the best approach.

Dr. Hamby also suggests that we need to ensure that our research and the results of the research are adapted for specific cultural groups and communities. While we may find that a specific curriculum is effective in inner city New York, that same curriculum may be ineffective in a rural area. Research needs to address cultural issues in prevention programming. Dr. Hamby also makes a case for including factors such as attendance, program integrity, and facilitator skill in our analyses. She makes a strong case for studies, such as the one proposed by Finkelhor and colleagues in 1988, that compare different types of programs and that follow participants over time to see how the programming impacts the future rate of IPV among participants.

O'Leary, Woodin, and Fritz also offer suggestions for future research in the area of IPV prevention programming. They encourage new researchers to be aware of the problems inherent in evaluating prevention programs. They suggest that ceiling effects can keep researchers from being able to measure program effectiveness. If programs are offered to all students in a grade, most of them will already have reasonable attitudes about more extreme forms of dating violence at pre-test. Therefore, it will be difficult to find significant changes unless the programs are targeted to high-risk youth. While they recognize limitations with targeted prevention programs, they encourage researchers to consider the problem of ceiling effects in designing studies.

O'Leary and colleagues also emphasize the importance of measuring not only attitude change, but also behavior change. They encourage researchers to use multi-method (interview and self-report), multi-respondent (self and partner) approaches whenever possible. Furthermore, they recommend that researchers evaluate separate components within their overall programs. Finally, they make a strong case for the importance of long-term follow-up. We need to have a better understanding of the long-term effects of dating violence prevention programming.

Dr. Suggs makes a case for a large research agenda regarding best practices in diagnosing and intervening with partner violence in the medical setting. She encourages researchers to develop and test a variety of short, valid, and reliable assessment instruments for IPV to be used with different patient populations and practice sites. She suggests that physicians would be much more likely to use a one or two item scale for universal screening than the longer scales currently available. Next, she suggests that qualitative studies using focus groups and key informants are needed to develop culturally appropriate interventions the provider can use when a partner violence victim is identified. She also suggests that once the intervention is formulated and outcomes defined, longitudinal, randomized control trials of the intervention need to occur. We need evidence that screening tools and health care provider interventions are effective in reducing future violence. She also advocates for research to determine how to teach medical providers about partner violence and partner violence screening. She suggests we need research to determine the most cost effective, efficient, and efficacious intervention that improves providers' practices with partner violence.

Hamberger and Phelan, in their examination of research on overcoming barriers to screening, identifying, and helping partner violence victims, suggest that more large, representative sample surveys need to be conducted with specific medical specialties and disciplines and work settings. They suggest that conclusions drawn from studying family physicians may not generalize to obstetricians, and so on. They also make a case for better survey research and more research to identify mechanisms by which various barriers inhibit screening. They also emphasize the importance of culturally relevant research when attempting to identify barriers to screening and intervening with abuse victims in medical settings because of racial disparities in health care access. They advocate for experimental studies to assist us in developing conclusions about the impact and value of written protocols and chart prompts for increasing screening behavior and identification of abuse in medical settings. Hamberger and Phelan echo the concern expressed by Suggs that no data exists that documents how health care screening and interventions developed by medical personnel impact the lives of abuse victims who are identified in medical settings. Clearly, the impact of health care interventions with abused women is one of the major research gaps in this area.

Campbell and Manganello suggest that a large research agenda also exists in the area of changing public attitudes to prevent IPV. There are few studies that even address interventions aimed to influence public perceptions about the issue. While campaigns to change public attitudes have been effective in a number of health-related areas, such as seat-belt campaigns and encouraging health care screening, we know very little about the effectiveness of public awareness campaigns in preventing partner violence. The studies that have been conducted in the area have many limitations. Campbell and Manganello recommend that we need better evaluation of campaigns and better definition of outcome variables and measurement of these outcomes. It is also important to have a comparison group that does not receive the media campaign in order to attribute the changes to a campaign. They end their article suggesting that, "In order for us to know if these campaigns are effective and what components should be replicated, rigorous, well-designed and funded evaluations are also necessary" (p. 34).

Wray supports the ideas presented by Campbell and Manganello and argues strongly that theory is an essential underpinning for intervention design and assessment. He suggests that without clear and explicit theories guiding communication interventions to prevent interpersonal violence, we are unable to explore our assumptions and make them explicit, analyze problems systematically, devise reasonable goals, or unify program planning and evaluation design. He further suggests that the reach of a campaign is directly related to its potential for success. He advocates for increased research on how to disseminate messages. He suggests we must develop and test theory-based mechanisms for intimate violence prevention and continue to explore avenues for gaining maximal exposure and accounting for multiple levels of influence. Finally, he cites the work of Hornik (2002) and suggests that researchers seeking to evaluate the impact of communication interventions incorporate measurement at multiple time points, compare exposed and unexposed populations, establish that effects are consistent with theoretical models, triangulate evidence, and focus on audience segments.

Finally, Mancini, Nelson, Bowen, and Martin, in their article examining a community capacity approach to preventing IPV, emphasize the lack of research connecting community dimensions with IPV. They suggest the need for a comprehensive community-based research approach that would account for the multiple layers of community that may influence people's engagement in the community and in prevention activities. Furthermore, they suggest that a primary research question would tease apart elements of community life and examine the role of various elements of community life in either mitigating or exacerbating partner violence. They advocate for research that examines the relationship between formal and informal networks of social care. They suggest that we need studies addressing how formal networks engage informal networks in prevention activities and how the informal networks contribute to their viability. They also make a case for research examining how community elements compare with other factors in explaining, understanding, and predicting partner violence and recommend comparative studies that examine the role of community in extreme groups. Groups high in partner violence can be compared with groups low in partner violence to determine the nature of community connections in these groups. Finally, they advocate for systematic evaluation of coordinated community responses and other community collaborations designed to prevent IPV. They suggest that unless systematic evaluations are conducted, such programs are "intentions-based rather than science-based" (p. 224).

The conclusion I draw from the manuscripts in this volume is that an extensive research agenda urgently awaits creative funding mechanisms and innovative research teams. Some of studies most urgently needed include:

1. Longitudinal, randomized clinical trials that test the effectiveness of various interventions in actually preventing IPV.
2. Studies that assist us in developing and testing theory to guide prevention interventions.
3. Studies to determine how to screen and intervene to prevent partner violence in health care settings.
4. Studies to determine how to train and motivate medical personnel to use screening tools and protocols.
5. Careful, controlled studies to determine the most effective content, format, and delivery methods for public awareness and media campaigns to prevent IPV.
6. Better evaluation of public awareness campaigns and better definition of outcome variables and measurement of these outcomes.
7. Studies that include a strong cost-benefit analysis so that when decision-makers are choosing interventions, they know how these interventions compare with alternative interventions.
8. Studies that assist us in developing prevention interventions for specific cultural groups and that allow us to assess the effectiveness of prevention interventions within various cultural groups.
9. Studies that assess how community collaborations impact the rate of IPV.

REFERENCES

Finkelhor, D., Hotaling, G. T., & Yllo, K. (1988). *Stopping family violence: Research priorities in the coming decade.* Newbury Park, CA: Sage.
Hornik, R. (Ed). (2002). *Public health communication: Evidence for behavior change.* Mahwah, NJ: Lawrence Erlbaum.

doi:10.1300/J146v13n03_09

APPENDIX

Prevention Programs Work Group	Health/Mental Health Screening Work Group	Public Awareness Work Group
Karen Rosen, Ed.D. **Group Facilitator** Associate Professor, Human Development, Virginia Tech	**Eric McCollum, Ph.D.** **Group Facilitator** Professor and Clinical Director, Human Development, Virginia Tech	**Marilyn Keel** **Group Facilitator** Program Analyst, Family Advocacy Program, ODASD (MC&FP)
Daniel O'Leary, Ph.D. Distinguished Professor, Department of Psychology, SUNY at Stony Brook	**Kevin Hamberger, Ph.D.** Professor, Family & Community Medicine, Medical College of Wisconsin	**Jackie Campbell, Ph.D., RN** Assoc. Dean of Doctoral Education Programs and Research, School of Nursing, Johns Hopkins University
Sherry Hamby, Ph.D. Director, Possible Equalities, Laurinburg, NC	**Nancy Sugg, M.D., M.P.H.** Associate Professor, University of Washington	**Ricardo Wray, Ph.D.** Research Fellow, Center for Community-based Research, Dana Farber Cancer Institute, Harvard
COL Rene Robichaux USA Chief, Behavioral Health Division, US Army Medical Command	**CDR Kathy Dully USN** Dept of Emergency Medicine, Naval Medical Center San Diego	**Col John Nelson USAF** Chief, Family Advocacy Division, USAF Medical Operations Agency
CAPT Frances Stewart, USN Director, Patient Advocacy & Medical Ethics, OASD (HA)	**Gayle Wiggins** Defense Task Force on Domestic Violence	**LTC Jim Jackson USA** Defense Task Force on Domestic Violence
LTC Yvonne Tucker-Harris USA Deputy Director for Family Programs, Army Community and Family Support Center	**LTC Cameron Ritchie USA** Program Director, Mental Health Policy & Women's Health Policy, OASD (HA)	**LTC Mark Chapin USA** Director of Research, Dept. of Family Medicine, F. Edward Hebert School of Medicine, USUHS
Terri Rau, Ph.D. Counseling, Advocacy & Prevention Branch, Navy Personnel Command	**Felicia Cohn, Ph.D.** Director of Medical Ethics Education, UC-Irvine College of Medicine	**Lenore Walker, Ph.D.** Executive Director, Domestic Violence Institute, Ft. Lauderdale, FL
Ed McCarroll, Ph.D. Professor, Dept. of Psychiatry, F. Edward Hebert School of Medicine, USUHS	**Col Martha Louis Davis USA** F Director, Family Advocacy Program, Air Force Medical Support Agency	**Mike Hoskins** Head, Counseling, Advocacy & Prevention Branch, Navy Personnel Command
Vickii Coffey Senior Advisor, Institute on Domestic Violence in the African American Community	**Elaine Woodhouse** Family Advocacy Program, Marine Corps Headquarters	**Mary Page** Manpower and Reserve Affairs, Marine Corps Headquarters
Lisa Schultz Program Manager, Axiom Resource Management, Inc.	**Rosemary Smith** Family Advocacy Program Manager, Defense Logistics Agency	**Bill Riley** Director, Family Violence Prevention & Services, Admin. For Children & Families, HHS

APPENDIX (continued)

Prevention Programs Work Group	Health/Mental Health Screening Work Group	Public Awareness Work Group
Bob Geffner, Ph.D. Family Violence & Sexual Assault Institute, Alliant International University	**Ileana Arias, Ph.D.** Chief, Etiology & Surveillance Branch, Nat'l Center for Injury Prevention and Control, CDC	**Leora Rosen, Ph.D.** Senior Social Science Analyst, Office of Research and Evaluation, NIJ
Maj Mike Zeliff USMC Defense Task Force on Domestic Violence	**Mary Hancock Stewart, MD** American College of Emergency Physicians	**Joel Milner, Ph.D.** Director, Center for the Study of Family Violence & Sexual Assault, NIU
	LtCol Deborah Bostock USAF Director, University Health Center, Dept. of Family Medicine, USUHS	**Janet Carter** Vice President, Family Violence Prevention Fund, San Francisco
	Debbie Tucker Executive Director, National Training Center on Domestic and Sexual Violence, Austin, TX	**CAPT Glenna Tinney USN** Deputy Director, Defense Task Force on Domestic Violence

Floaters:
David Lloyd, Director, Family Advocacy Program, ODASD (MC&FP)

LtCol Dari Tritt USAF, Research Director, Family Advocacy Program, USAF Medival Operations Agency

Sandra M. Stith, PhD, Program Director, Family and Child Development, Department of Human Development, Virginia Tech

Index

T - #0502 - 101024 - C0 - 212/152/15 - PB - 9780789030337 - Gloss Lamination